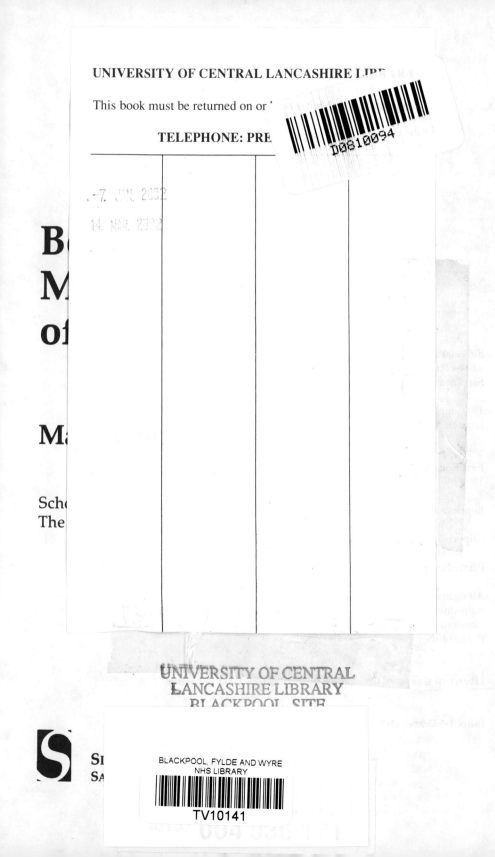

B

M

of

Ma

Sch
The

S

Si

SA

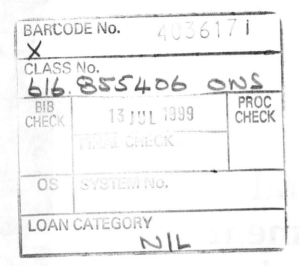
**Singular Publishing** Group, Inc.
4284 41st Street
San Diego, CA 92105-1197

19 Compton Terrace
London N1 2UN, United Kingdom


First Edition
1993 by Livingston Press, Sydney

Reprinted 1996 by Singular Publishing Group, Inc.

Copyright © 1996 by Singular Publishing Group

Printed in the United States of America by McNaughton and Gunn

**Library of Congress Cataloging-in-Publication Data available**


**ISBN 1-56593-633-7**

# Preface

This project began some years ago as sketchy notes for a two-semester undergraduate course at the School of Communication Disorders, The University of Sydney. The structure of the book reflects the content of that course. I am grateful to the many students and speech pathologists who supported and encouraged its development.

I feel that the influence of Roger Ingham is present in these pages, even though it is nearly ten years since his departure from the School of Communication Disorders. After the period of his influence, I was fortunate enough to work closely for a long period with Cheryl Andrews, Leanne Costa, and Elisabeth Harrison at the Lidcombe Hospital Stuttering Unit, and Ann Packman and Michelle Lincoln at the School of Communication Disorders. These people provided an environment which bristled with challenges and stimulation. Without them there would be no book. There also would be no book without Anne, Kate, and Joel, who, along with everything else, somehow managed to put up with me while I wrote it.

Ann Packman assisted me with organizing the material in Part Five. The section "Speech Motor Control" in Part Five was written with the assistance of Ann Packman, and the section "Anxiety" in Part Five was written with the assistance of Michelle Lincoln. The editorial input of Ann Packman and Elisabeth Harrison prevented me from causing too much damage to the English language.

With these expressions of gratitude comes the end of writing, also thankfully.

August 1993,
Sydney.

# Contents

# Part Three:
# Management of Early Stuttering

# Part Four:
# Management of Advanced Stuttering

# Part Five:
# Perspectives on Stuttering

# Part Six:
# Clinical Issues in Management of
# Advanced Stuttering

# Part Seven:
# Clinical Issues in Management of
# Early Stuttering

# Part Eight:
# Clinical Issues in Measurement of Stuttering

# Part One:

# Basic Information for Clinical Practice

# Describing Stuttering

## Basic terminology

This is one way that stuttering could be described:

> It is a disorder where speech disruptions occur and may interfere with normal communication. Most of these speech disruptions are repetitions of sounds or syllables, prolongations of sounds, or periods during which speech production is "blocked." Verbal disruptions may be accompanied by nonverbal events such as grimacing, blinking or other facial movements.

The terms "stuttering" and "stammering" refer to the same disorder, although the latter term is rarely used outside the United Kingdom. One of the most influential ideas about the condition is that it consists of moments of stuttering which occur in otherwise normal speech. This idea is a clinically useful one that has gained widespread acceptance by clinicians. It is also quite controversial, and is discussed in detail in Part Eight.

A moment of stuttering can be referred to as a "stutter," a "moment of stuttering," a "stuttering moment," or a "stuttering." The terms "disfluency" "dysfluency," and "nonfluency" are often used to refer to a moment of stuttering. However, this practice can cause confusion because those terms are used sometimes to describe normal speech disruptions that are not part of stuttering. Finn and Ingham (1989) have pointed out that "disfluency" is a better term for normal speech disruptions than "dysfluency" because the prefix "dys" means "abnormal," and so the term "normal dysfluency" is intrinsically contradictory. In this text the term "stutter" is used to refer to a moment of stuttering, and "normal disfluency" is used to refer to a speech disruption which is not part of stuttering. The term "disfluency" is used as a general reference to "stuttering" and "normal disfluency."

Speech that is perceived not to contain stuttering can be referred to as "stutter-free speech." The terms "fluent" and "fluency" are often used to mean "stutter-free speech," although in a sense they are awkward because they refer to everything that is not stuttering. Such terminology does not occur in the management of other disorders. For example, those who treat clients for chain smoking have no need for a term that includes everything that is not smoking. Finn and Ingham (1989) have drawn attention to another problem with the terms "fluent" and "fluency." These terms are commonly used to refer to several dimensions of speech and language. To say that a person is a fluent speaker does not necessarily mean that the person does not stutter. For example, someone can be said to be "fluent" in a second language. Hence it is not clear what is meant by "fluent" and "fluency" or their opposites "disfluent" or "disfluency."

A recent development in terminology is the "person first" way of referring to those who stutter. This is referring to a person who has a disorder rather than using the name of the disorder to refer to the person. So, the term "stutterer" could be replaced with "person who stutters," "client who stutters," "someone who stutters," and so on. The American Speech-Language-Hearing Association, which publishes international journals including the Journal of Speech and Hearing Research and the American Journal of Speech-Language Pathology, encourages its authors to use "person first" references to those who have communication disorders.[1]

# Verbal features

The most common verbal features of the disorder are multiple repetitions of the first sound or syllable in a word, prolongations of sounds, and "blocks" in the progress of speech, during which the speaker may seem to be struggling. Blocks can be debilitating speech disruptions, and in severe cases may last for as long as 30 seconds. Other kinds of stuttering are repetitions of whole words of one or more syllables, interjections such as "um" and "you see," phrase repetitions, revisions, interjections, restarts, and phrase repetitions.[2] These different kinds of stuttering behaviors are *not necessarily mutually exclusive*. Stuttered speech is a complex thing, and any given stutter might be described with more than one of the terms above. For example, a prolongation and a repetition of a word can happen at the same time. Onslow, Gardner, Bryant, Stuckings, and Knight (1992) showed that clinicians may use up to five different terms to describe some disfluencies.

# Nonverbal features

These do not always occur, but when they do they can be the most disfiguring features of the disorder. They include body, head and facial movements such as head jerking, tongue protrusion, twitching, blinking, and movements of limbs or torso. Nonverbal features occur concurrently with verbal features. Head, facial, and other movements are as much a part of a moment of stuttering as are the verbal features discussed above. This means that if no verbal features are heard but head, body or facial movements are observed, a clinician may judge that a stutter has occurred.

The fact that stuttering may involve nonverbal features has two clinical implications. The first — and the most important — is that a clinician needs to *look at as well as listen to the client* in order to be absolutely sure that stuttered speech is not present. As discussed in many places in this text, audio tape recorders are extremely useful in stuttering treatment. However, it is worth remembering that a clinician's detection of stuttered speech from an audio tape recording may not be as reliable as when the clinician can see the client speaking. Some clients have stuttered speech which is difficult to detect on an audio tape recording. The second clinical implication of body, head and facial movements in stuttering is that similar movements occur in various tic syndromes (Turpin, 1983). Particularly in the case of young children, tics may resemble stuttering to some extent. It does not happen often, but tics and stuttering in young children can be confused.

Some people who stutter may experience negative emotions in connection with the disorder. Some examples are fear or anxiety about speaking, lack of social or professional confidence, and frustration. Occasionally, these emotions can be more disabling than stuttered speech itself. For example, clients have been known to have serious anxiety attacks if they are required to answer a telephone. However, on the whole, people who stutter cope well with, what can be, a debilitating disorder. In fact, there are many people who stutter and choose to live with the condition. Such people may find that it is a nuisance at times, but

---

[1] However, it is clear at present what those who stutter think about the term "stutterer."

[2] The terms "tense pause" and "dysrhythmic phonation" are used in the research literature. It is not completely clear, but the former term is probably a synonym for "block," and the latter probably is a synonym for "prolongation."

are able to communicate adequately and do not experience negative emotions about their speech.

An important nonverbal feature of the disorder is word avoidance. Some clients are skilled at scanning forward while speaking and avoiding words on which they are likely to stutter. Such strategies include circumlocution and word substitution. If these strategies are successful, stuttering can be exposed in speaking situations in which words cannot be avoided. Examples of such situations include reading out loud, reciting set material in public, and placing an order in a restaurant. Word avoidance is a particular concern for clinicians because it can be difficult to detect.

# Defining Stuttering

It is an interesting exercise to observe normal speech for a while and then look again at the description of stuttering on page 12. It is obvious that many of the terms that can be used to describe stuttered speech can also be used to describe anyone's speech. For example, all speakers experience speech "disruptions" which might be described as "repetitions" or "blockages." These terms therefore cannot be used to distinguish between normal speech events and the speech events of stuttering.

When describing the disorder of stuttering, these limitations of terminology are not a great concern. But defining the disorder is something different. A definition of stuttering is more than a description because it must present criteria which an observer can use to distinguish stuttered speech from nonstuttered speech. Also, the observer should be able to use a definition to decide whether a speech event such as a "repetition" or a "prolongation" is normal or is part of the disorder.

Clinicians stand to benefit from having a definition of stuttering. A definition would let a clinician know exactly which "repetitions," "prolongations," and so on, should be counted as part of stuttering and which should not be counted because they are a part of normal speech. More importantly, a definition would help clinicians decide who has the disorder and who has not. This is not an issue for adults and children who have been stuttering for some years. Obviously, if it is a problem for them, they—or their parents in the case of children—will present themselves to a clinic. However one aspect of stuttering management considered in great detail in this text is that clinicians need to treat the disorder when the first signs of it appear in young children. In order to do that, clinicians need a definition of what those first signs are.

Unfortunately, defining stuttering is not a straightforward matter. There is no definition that everyone agrees on, only a number of viewpoints about the matter. In the following sections, three such viewpoints are considered, along with the strengths and limitations of each.

## Symptomatic definition

A symptomatic definition involves a list of observable features of the disorder. The potential benefit of symptomatic definition is that independent observers could use it to determine who does and who does not stutter, and also to determine whether certain speech features are a part of stuttering or a part of normal speech. There are many symptomatic definitions of stuttering available, but probably the most popular is that offered by Wingate (1964):

> (a) Disruption in the fluency of verbal expression, which (b) is characterized by involuntary, audible or silent, repetitions or prolongations in the utterance of short speech elements, namely: sound, syllables and words of one syllable. The disruptions (c) usually occur frequently or are marked in character and (d) are not readily controllable. (p. 488)

Another symptomatic definition appears in the World Health Organization's (1977) International Classification of Diseases:

Disorders in the rhythm of speech, in which the individual knows precisely what he wishes to say, but at the time is unable to say it because of an involuntary, repetitive prolongation or cessation of a sound. (p. 202)

Ingham (1984) has noted that one difficulty with Wingate's definition, which also applies to the World Health Organization definition, is that it contains "qualifiers and imprecise terms" (p. 17), such as "fluency," "usually," "readily," and "short." To that might be added that "involuntary" and "controllable" are speech dimensions that cannot be observed, and therefore they are of limited use as part of a symptomatic definition. For example, if one observer said that a certain speech disruption was "involuntary" and another observer said that it was "voluntary," it would be difficult to resolve the difference.

Another problem with symptomatic definitions is that stuttering is not a straightforward set of speech events. People do a lot of complicated things when they stutter. Also, stuttering differs a great deal among people who are affected by it. In fact, just about everyone who stutters has something unique about their stuttering. In short, it is difficult to imagine any symptomatic definition of stuttering that embraces all the speech perturbations of all people who have the condition.

On the other hand, it may not be necessary to include all the diverse speech events of stuttering within a definition. It might be that all people who stutter have some of the same speech events, and that these events can be used to define the disorder. Following this line of reasoning, Andrews, Craig, Feyer, Hoddinott, Howie and Neilson (1983), have asserted that "repetitions and prolongations are necessary and sufficient for the diagnosis of stuttering" (p. 227). But this symptomatic definition, along with all others that have been suggested, fails to distinguish effectively between stuttered and normal speech. Things that may be described as "repetitions and prolongations" happen when anyone speaks—perhaps not all the time, but they certainly happen. So it is a problem if they alone are used to determine whether or not a person stutters.

## Internal definition

Perkins (1984a) offers a definition of stuttering that incorporates the idea that stuttering is a private event, and as such is unavailable for objective scrutiny: "Temporary overt or covert loss of control of the ability to move forward fluently in the execution of linguistically formulated speech" (p. 431).[1] Perkins' definition implies that only those with the disorder can determine whether stuttering is present or absent. Moore and Perkins (1990) reported an experiment where a subject spoke with real and faked stuttering. They reported that the speaker could tell the difference between the two, but observers could not. This "internal" perspective on defining stuttering certainly has some valid aspects. Few would argue that one way to find out if a person stutters is to ask that person. Similarly, one way to find out whether a certain speech event is a part of stuttering is to ask the speaker.

Although an internal definition has merit because of its validity, it has some serious shortcomings. As with symptomatic definitions, it fails to distinguish between speech which does and does not contain stuttering. Obviously, there are occasions when all speakers lose control of the ability to "move forward fluently." Another problem is that defining stuttering as a completely private event makes it inaccessible to observers. Martin and Haroldson (1986) have argued that this limits the usefulness of the definition in scientific research. However, clinicians could rely on their clients to tell them when stuttering occurs. But as

---

[1] Siegel (1987) has made an interesting comment about Perkins' definition. It is more than a definition; it is a theoretical statement about the nature of the disorder.

Perkins (1990a) himself notes, this is not a practical basis for identifying stuttering in young children; even if adults can reliably distinguish between being "in control" and "out of control," it is doubtful that young children could do the same.

## Consensus definition

Bloodstein (1987) suggests that stuttering could be defined as "whatever is perceived as stuttering by a reliable observer who has relatively good agreement with others" (p. 9). The argument is that a consensus, made up of the perceptions of experienced people in a clinical community, should determine what stuttering is and is not. The consensus definition is a perceptual one. In other words, stuttering is defined in terms of whether or not observers think it is present. There is some appeal in this notion because, on most occasions at least, it seems that stuttered speech is readily perceptible.

An often cited criticism of this approach is that it is not "objective." If two observers think that speech contains stuttering, it is not necessarily known what features of speech caused the observers to think that. The identifying features of the stuttered speech cannot be written down for use by another observer. The concept of consensus definition may also be criticized because its procedures are not clear. What is the meaning of "reliable" and "relatively good agreement with others," and how should it be determined that a given observer possesses these attributes? Who are the "others" with whom the observer should agree? Should observers who are "unreliable" and without "agreement with others" be trained, or should they be excluded from judging the presence of the disorder? And if they are to be trained, what should be the training procedures?

## Defining stuttering in clinical practice

Many of the issues above, and more, have been discussed at length by scholars and researchers for a decade as they have searched for a satisfactory definition of stuttering (Bloodstein, 1990; Ingham, 1990a; Martin & Haroldson, 1986; Moore & Perkins, 1990; Perkins, 1983a; 1984a; 1986; 1990a; 1990b; Smith, 1990; Wingate, 1984). This body of literature conveys the impression that there may never be general agreement about how to define stuttering. This sends the important message to clinicians that defining stuttering is not a straightforward matter, and a simplistic and inflexible approach to it will not suffice.

Bloodstein (1990) notes that different clinical situations call for different definitions. For example, a clinician might require a client to monitor for the occurrence of stuttering throughout each day. Obviously, in such a case, an internal definition would be a suitable choice. On the other hand, a clinician might wish to provide information to the public about the disorder, in which case a symptomatic definition might be the most suitable. A situation that occurs many times in day-to-day clinical practice is that clients attempt to speak without stuttering while the clinician listens and gives feedback about whether stuttering has or has not occurred. In such situations a consensus definition might be the most suitable; stuttering is deemed to have occurred if the clinician, who has agreement with other clinicians, perceives that it has. A later section considers in detail a particularly important situation in clinical practice where a definition of stuttering is required. That situation is when the clinician has to diagnose whether or not a young child has begun to stutter.

# Epidemiology of Stuttering

Epidemiology is the study of rates of diseases in populations and the variables that influence those rates. There are many ways that clinicians can make use of epidemiological information about stuttering. Andrews (1984a) states that it can provide information which is valuable in determining the cause of a disorder and how it should be treated. Epidemiological data about stuttering can contribute to understanding its nature and etiology, because explanations of its cause and nature must be consistent with those data (as well as with everything else that is known about it). Epidemiological information about stuttering can be important in the planning of health care services for it. For example, the number of people in an urban region who stutter might be cited as a justification for the employment of a clinician who specializes in stuttering management. Even more important is knowledge about the untreated course of the disorder. Does the condition worsen with time, or might recovery be expected? If untreated, is the disorder likely to cause significant human distress or to affect quality of life? It is essential for clinicians to provide information about the untreated course of the disorder, so that clients (or their parents) can make an informed decision about whether to undertake treatment. Such information is particularly important in the case of children who have just begun to stutter. Should treatment begin immediately, or should the parent wait for a certain period of time in the hope that the disorder will remit? What risks would be involved in delaying the onset of treatment? Do the ill effects of the disorder on young children justify the inconvenience of the treatment?[1]

Stuttering is one of many communication disorders. Comparing its features to other disorders can provide information which is useful for making decisions about service delivery: How common is it compared to other speech/language disorders? What is the extent of suffering that it causes relative to those other disorders? Is it distinctive because of urgent needs for treatment at onset or during a certain period of its development? This information is relevant to the making of certain clinical decisions. Should children who have recently begun to stutter be given waiting list priority? What portion of available clinician time in a clinic should be directed to the management of stuttering clients? When clients have one or more communication disorders in addition to stuttering, should treatment priority be given to one disorder?

There is much information about the nature of stuttering that is conveyed by epidemiological data, and that information is useful when describing the nature of the disorder to clients. Clients who stutter, or parents or spouses of stuttering clients, need to know the nature of the speech problem. Useful information in such a context includes how common stuttering is, the patterns of its onset and remission, and the way it develops from early childhood through to adulthood.

---

[1] These issues are considered in detail in Part Seven.

# Prevalence

Prevalence refers to the number of cases of a disease in a population at a given time. In the case of stuttering, Bloodstein (1987) shows that studies have yielded a consistent result of around 1 percent prevalence for stuttering. Andrews (1984a) remarks that, therefore, it is not a rare disorder.

# Incidence

Incidence refers to the number of new cases of a disease that occur in a given period of time. Lifetime incidence is a figure that depicts the proportion of a population ever to have a disorder. It is generally accepted that the lifetime incidence of stuttering is higher than its prevalence. The likely reason for this is that, as discussed later, stuttering is particularly tractable in the first years after onset, and so efforts to treat it are likely to be extremely successful in those early years. Bloodstein (1987) concludes from his review of the literature the lifetime incidence of stuttering is 4 to 5 percent.

# Onset

Information about the age at which stuttering begins should be treated with some caution because it is mostly gathered from the recall of parents, which may not be accurate owing to the time elapsed since onset. Another reason parent recall data may be unreliable is that a child may be stuttering for some time before parents notice (Bloodstein, 1987). These problems have been offset somewhat by recent studies involving parent interviews quite soon after onset (Yairi, 1983; Yairi & Ambrose, 1992a).[1] Bloodstein (1987) reviews survey data about the onset of stuttering and concludes that "the earliest age of onset of stuttering is quite consistently recalled as about eighteen months" (p. 92). The latest age of onset in these data ranges from 7 to 13 years.

The data summarized by Bloodstein (p. 93) provide several reasons to think that stuttering begins mostly in the first few years of life. First, the recalled mean and median age of onset generally is below 5 years. Second, the distribution of onset appears to be skewed. Bloodstein notes that mean age of onset in studies is generally closer to the earliest age of onset than to the latest age of onset. Third, some past and recent studies have consistently reported stuttering to have begun in the second and third year of life (Darley, 1955; Johnson, 1942; Johnson & Associates, 1959; Onslow, Harrison, & Jones, 1993; Yairi, 1983; Yairi & Ambrose, 1992a).

It appears from surveys of parents that a number of cases start quite suddenly. Yairi (1983) and Yairi and Ambrose (1992a) reported that, in just under half of cases, stuttering appeared in less than 1 week, with the remainder taking from 2 to 6 weeks, and sometimes longer. Those studies reported quite high proportions of children who began stuttering in one day; 36.4 percent for the former and 31.0 percent for the latter study. Onslow, Harrison, and Jones (1993) reported that 23 percent of parents said that their children's stuttering began in less than one week, with 4 percent of cases reportedly beginning in one day. Most parents in the latter category reported that their child's stuttering began "overnight." Clinicians sometimes encounter parents who state that their child went to bed speaking normally and was stuttering at breakfast time. In addition to beginning quickly, stuttering

---

[1] However, a problem incurred by such studies is that they may underestimate age of onset simply because they deal with younger subjects.

may also be quite severe soon after onset, and may be accompanied by head and facial movements (Conture & Kelly, 1991; Onslow, Harrison, & Jones, 1993; Yairi, 1983; Yairi, Ambrose, & Niermann, 1993; Yairi & Lewis, 1984). This information is important because it contradicts some influential, traditional views of stuttering onset as a gradual process. Those views are considered in Parts Five and Seven.

There are recurring suggestions in the literature that a subgroup of children begin to stutter after some kind of traumatic episode, which may be speech related (for example, Starkweather, 1987; Van Riper, 1971). However, Poulos and Webster (1991) reported some data which suggest that only a small number of cases may begin in this way. They found that of 169 adult and adolescents who stuttered, only three subjects reported episodes involving "intense fear" which might have precipitated stuttering.

It is generally accepted that a small number of cases begin in adulthood. Adult onset mostly occurs with accompanying neurological damage such as head injury or stroke (see Helm-Estabrooks, 1993; Rosenbek, 1984). Late onset cases not accompanied by neurological damage are sometimes reported as psychogenic in origin (For example, Mahr & Leith, 1992; Roth, Aronson, & Davis, 1989). Sometimes the terms "acquired" and "idiopathic" stuttering are used to distinguish developmental onset from onset related to neurological disturbance. One problem associated with the literature which describes adult-onset stuttering is that it is not clear whether subjects are stuttering or have some other speech change associated with neurological damage; for example, palilalia (La Point & Horner, 1981).

Case reports sometimes indicate stuttering onset in late childhood or early adulthood without accompanying trauma of any kind. It is conceivable in such cases that extremely mild and clinically insignificant stuttering was present in early childhood but was not recognized. It is possible for such stuttering to worsen and become clinically significant when more demands are placed on speech during adolescence and young adulthood. For example, a child may be enrolled in a school where speaking in front of class or school assembly is required, or a young adult may undertake a career which requires high-level verbal skills. It is possible that such stresses may bring extremely mild stuttering to clinically significant levels.

## "Spontaneous recovery"

In the past, clinical practice with young children who stutter has been dominated by a belief that around 80 percent of them do not require treatment because they recover from the disorder spontaneously. According to Martin and Lindamood (1986) that impression emerged in the 1960s from the results of a series of surveys (Martyn & Sheehan, 1968; Sheehan & Martyn, 1966; 1970) and from a longitudinal study of stuttering children by Andrews and Harris (1964). However, there have been several challenges to this notion in recent years. It now is generally accepted that the 80 percent estimate is far too high (Ingham, 1983; Martin & Lindamood, 1986; Wingate, 1976; Young, 1975a), and that the correct figure may be less than 50 percent. A recent longitudinal report by Ramig (1993) confirmed this possibility. Ramig reassessed 21 children 6 to 8 years after they were diagnosed as stuttering. Five of those children were younger than 5 years at diagnosis. Those children did not receive treatment at the time of diagnosis, and all five were found to be stuttering 6 to 8 years later.

Another important challenge to the notion of "spontaneous recovery" is studies which suggest that parents are likely to assist their children at the onset of stuttering (Andrews & Harris, 1964; Dickson, 1971; Glasner & Rosenthal, 1957; Johnson & Associates, 1959; Lankford & Cooper, 1974; Onslow, Harrison & Jones, 1993). In many cases parents seem to do this by saying things when their children stutter such as "stop and start again," and "slow down." As stated in many places in this text, there is every reason to believe that such actions will help eliminate stuttering. Ingham (1983) reviewed the "spontaneous recovery" research, and concluded that

> for many stutterers a program of specific speech modification, constantly managed and associated with substantial practice, probably aids recovery and is largely responsible for "spontaneous remission." The self-assisting aids that adult subjects claim to use with success are also frequently advocated by the parents of many children who stutter. (p. 132)

The issue of recovery from stuttering without clinic attendance is one which clinicians need to consider in detail, because it has important implications for the provision of treatment services. Consequently, the topic is resumed and considered in more detail in Part Seven.

## The role of genetics

One of the most useful pieces of epidemiological information about stuttering is that, to some extent, genetics influences who will develop it. However, the details about this are not yet clear (Kidd, 1984; Pauls, 1990). Around one half to two thirds of stuttering clients report that they have a relative affected with the disorder. This means that a person who stutters has more chance than a nonstuttering person of having a child who stutters. The clinical implications of this are that the children of people who stutter should be monitored for early signs of the disorder. Genetics and stuttering are considered in more detail in Part Five.

## The sex ratio

Stuttering affects more males than females, with reported ratios varying from 3:1 to 5:1. Many clinicians believe that not only fewer girls begin to stutter, but those who do are much more prone to recovery than boys. One problem in interpreting the sex ratio is that there are other communication disorders of childhood (such as phonological and language impairment) which affect males more than females. Consequently, it is not clear whether the male/female ratio of stuttering reflects something about stuttering or something about all speech and language disorders.

# Speaking Conditions That Reduce Stuttering

It is well known that many speaking conditions can reduce stuttering severity. In the short term, the effects of all these conditions are transitory; stuttering will be reduced or eliminated when the conditions are present, only to reappear as soon as, or shortly after, they are removed. Some of these speaking conditions can be adapted for use as treatment techniques, some are useful accessories to treatment, and some are important to know about because they can interact with treatments. Many of these conditions have been researched extensively. The purpose of this section is to briefly describe these speaking conditions and to note their clinical relevance. Where appropriate, details about their clinical application and research about them are presented in later sections. Ingham (1984) and Wingate (1976) give an account of all the conditions mentioned below, and this section draws freely from those sources.

The material presented in the following sections is puzzling, because it shows that there are many ways of speaking that can reduce stuttering. Van Riper (1971) has remarked how frustrating it can be for a clinician that so many things can reduce stuttering so well but so briefly. Wingate (1969; 1970) raised the notion that all these speaking conditions can reduce stuttering because they have something in common. Wingate suggested that the thing in common is a change in "vocal expression." In other words, if someone who stutters changes their "vocal expression," this is likely to modify stuttering. This is the "modified vocalization hypothesis."

## Delayed auditory feedback/prolonged speech

Delayed auditory feedback involves use of an apparatus which slightly delays the arrival of sidetone (the speaker's airborne speech signal) to the speaker's ears. This may cause the speaker to adopt an unusual speech pattern, presumably in an effort to overcome the effects of the delay. Goldiamond (1965) discovered that this speech pattern can eliminate stuttered speech, and coined the term "prolonged speech" to describe it. Prolonged speech has profoundly influenced stuttering treatments, being the basis of the most commonly used treatment for adults who stutter. A less important influence of DAF arose from observations that, with normal speakers, it may cause disruptions which bear a superficial resemblance to stuttering. This prompted the formulation of theories which suggest that the cause of stuttering is disturbed auditory feedback. Prolonged speech treatments and DAF theories of the cause of stuttering will be considered in detail in later sections.

## Masking

This term describes the use of noise (usually white noise) to impair a person's hearing of sidetone. In the case of people who stutter, masking may reduce stuttering. A body-worn device, called the Edinburgh Masker, is designed to reduce stuttering by activating a masking noise during speech. The client wears earphones and a small microphone attached to the neck over the larynx. Whenever the client speaks, this is detected by the microphone and the masking noise in the earphones is activated. A study reported by Block and Ingham (1983) suggested that there is little clinical value in this device. With 14 subjects, stuttering was reduced on average around 50 percent, and stuttering was not completely eliminated for any subject.

## Adaptation

Generally, after five consecutive readings of the same material, stuttering severity will be reduced by around 50 percent. This effect is called adaptation, and it is one of the most researched aspects of stuttering. Yet it is an effect which seems to be of little use to clinicians. This is because a stuttering reduction of 50 percent is not clinically significant on most occasions, and the effect does not continue when a person ceases to read and resumes conversational speech. Nonetheless, it is worth noting that a treatment procedure that involves repeated reading of material may reduce stuttering because of adaptation rather than because of the effects of the treatment.

## Rhythmic stimulation

This is probably the best known and most effective condition for reducing stuttering. Rhythmic speech may have been used as a treatment for stuttering in the third century BC. In the earlier part of this century, rhythmic speech was the basis for many popular but dubious therapy practices where clients paid considerable amounts to learn to speak in rhythm as a treatment for their stuttering (Clark, 1964). Rhythmic speech reappeared in a more respectable guise in the 1960s, with the development of "syllable-timed speech" programs. This kind of rhythmic speech involves saying each syllable in time to a rhythmic beat. A metronome was a common therapy aid in this form or treatment, and some body-worn metronome devices were made to deliver auditory or vibrotactile stimulation. Rhythmic stimulation can be auditory, visual, or vibrotactile. The effects of rhythmic speech highlight one of the most problematic aspects of managing stuttering that will be considered many times in this text; although rhythmic speech may be stutter-free, it sounds far from normal.

## Altered prosody

Imitating an accent, or otherwise altering customary prosodic patterns, may eliminate or reduce stuttering. This may be the reason why actors who stutter have been known to be free of the problem when performing. Another interesting report is that, for some people, stuttering is virtually eliminated when they are angry. The reason for this may be that anger changes customary prosody. Whispering is another speech mode which can reduce stuttering to some extent. Stuttering is nearly always eliminated during singing.

## Reduced speech rate

This effect is so well known that nearly all people who stutter report having received advice at some time to "slow down." Reduced speech rate often does reduce stuttering, however this strategy, alone, is unlikely to be a useful treatment for many clients. One reason for this is that the procedure does not necessarily eliminate all stuttering. Another reason is that it requires considerable effort to reduce speech rate habitually, and if the client is willing to undertake that much effort then some other treatment procedure is likely be a better choice. There are occasions, however, when speech rate modification is a satisfactory procedure. Those occasions will be discussed in a later section.

## Chorus reading and shadowing

Chorus reading is where the person who stutters reads aloud in unison with another person. The effect of this is for stuttering to disappear. The effect may be present to some extent when the accompanist does not read identical material, or even when the accompanist speaks nonsense syllables. The effect may be the result of reduced speech rate under chorus reading conditions, or to an alteration in prosody that occurs under those conditions. A related condition is shadowing, where the person who stutters repeats the utterances of a nonstuttering person as they are said. This reduces stuttering, although generally not as much as chorus reading. As with chorus reading, a likely explanation for the effect is that the condition involves a change of customary prosody.

# Early Stuttering

In this text the term "early stuttering" refers to children who have begun to stutter in the preschool years, most commonly in the second or third year of life, and who have been stuttering for a short period of from one to three years. Some clinicians use the term "incipient stuttering" in place of "early stuttering." In this text the term "advanced stuttering" refers to an adolescent or adult who has been stuttering since the preschool years. Some clinicians use the term "chronic stuttering" in place of "advanced stuttering."

## Studies describing normal disfluencies in early childhood

It is well known that all speakers, particularly preschool-age children, speak with some disfluencies. Wingate (1988) points out that there have been two research directions in this area. One research direction is with specific reference to stuttering and the other is without specific reference to stuttering. Wingate remarks that "the literature based in stuttering has remained insulated from the fairly extensive research on nonfluency in normal speech that has developed within the field of psycholinguistics" (p. 21). That field has researched speech events referred to as "hesitation phenomena."

Wingate points out a problem about terms, such as those on page 13, which are used to describe stuttered speech (blocks, prolongations, part-word repetitions, and so on). They have been used to compare the disfluencies of nonstuttering children with the disfluencies of stuttering children. But the terminology outlined on page 13 is not a proper way to describe the disfluencies of nonstuttering preschool children because, as discussed shortly, it was derived from a population of children where half of them stuttered. Wingate notes that many "hesitation phenomena" that might occur in young children's speech simply are not recorded with disfluency categories that are applied to stuttering research. This provides an important caveat to how we might interpret descriptions of normal disfluency based on disfluency terms; they likely are not a complete description at all. Wingate also comments that any measures of the disfluencies in normal speaking children is likely to be an underestimate simply because not all disfluencies are counted.

The above reservations considerably limit what can be concluded from studies of normal disfluency which use the disfluency categories outlined on page 13. It seems clear, though, from several studies (DeJoy & Gregory, 1985; Silverman, 1972; Yairi, 1981; 1982; Yairi & Clifton, 1972; Wexler & Mysak, 1982), that:

1. Disfluencies occur more in preschool children than older speakers.
2. The rate of disfluencies decreases during the preschool years.
3. Nonstuttering preschool children produce some speech events which can be described with the same terms used to describe speech events associated with stuttering children (see below); repetitions of parts of words, "tense pauses," and prolongations.

4. There is considerable variation in the disfluencies of early life. At different times, individual children will show considerable variability in the frequency of their disfluencies and in the predominance of various disfluency categories. Additionally, different children will show markedly different rates of disfluency.

# Studies of early stuttering

There is a body of literature which provides useful information about early stuttering. A detailed review of each of these studies is beyond the scope of this text. However, in the following sections the information contained in this literature is summarized.

## Verbal and nonverbal features

A number of studies have compared the speech of stuttering and nonstuttering children in order to identify speech features which characterize early stuttering.[1] Johnson and his colleagues at the University of Iowa published the results of a series of experiments that were conducted over a period of 20 years (Johnson & Associates, 1959), much of which concerned differences between early stuttering and normal disfluency. One part of this work involved speech measures on 68 stuttering and 68 normal children. The stuttering children showed significantly more repetitions, prolongations and "broken words." Additionally, the stuttering children were found to show significantly more "repetition units" per disfluency. The stuttering children showed a range of around one to three repetitions while nonstuttering children generally showed one to two repetition units.

Yairi and Lewis (1984) acquired speech samples from 10 stuttering children with a narrow age range (25-39 months, mean 29 months), and a short period from onset to data collection (mean of less than 2 months). Those speech samples were compared to those from 10 nonstuttering children. The rank order of frequency of disfluency for stuttering children was part-word repetition, dysrhythmic phonation, single-syllable word repetition; for the control children it was interjections, part-word repetition, revision-incomplete phrase. Repetition unit (RU) analysis showed a significant result for single-syllable word repetition (mean RU 1.34 compared with 1.09) and part-word repetition (mean RU 1.72 compared with 1.12). Nonstuttering children rarely exceeded 2 RUs, but for stuttering children the range was 1-11 RUs.

Several studies have reported that the disfluencies in nonstuttering preschool-age children and in early stuttering are not distributed randomly, but "cluster" together in sequences (Colburn, 1985; Hubbard & Yairi, 1988; Silverman, 1973). Hubbard and Yairi (1988) studied 15 stuttering and 15 nonstuttering preschool children (mean age 34 months). It was found that both stuttering and nonstuttering children's speech samples contained clustering of disfluencies at a level beyond that expected by chance. For the stuttering children there were significantly more clusters, and a significantly greater portion of disfluencies occurred in clusters. Size of clusters in the stuttering children ranged from two to 10 disfluencies, but only from two to five disfluencies in the nonstuttering subjects. Further, stuttering children had 40 percent of their clusters greater than two disfluencies, but nonstuttering children only had 19 percent of their clusters greater than two disfluencies. In

---

[1] Some studies have reported acoustic and physiological data about early stuttering (e.g. Adams, 1987; Conture, Rothenberg, & Molitar, 1986; Hall & Yairi, 1992), but the present discussion deals only with studies of clinically observable features.

the stuttering children, 18 percent of the clusters had four or more disfluencies, but only eight percent of the normal children's clusters had four or more disfluencies.

Zebrowski (1991) studied 10 stuttering and 10 nonstuttering children and found no significant differences between the groups for the durations of stutters or the number of RUs per disfluency. This finding contradicts that of Johnson and Associates (1959) and Yairi and Lewis (1984). It is of interest, however, that the Yairi and Lewis (1984) report studied children very soon after the onset of stuttering and reported a wide range of 1-11 repetitions in disfluencies. This raises the possibility that repetition units as a distinctive feature of early stuttering may occur soon after the onset of the disorder rather than at some later time. Zebrowski did find significant differences between the groups for the proportion of "sound/syllable repetitions" (part-word repetitions) and "audible sound prolongations."

In expanding on previous work (Schwartz, Zebrowski, & Conture, 1990; Schwartz & Conture, 1988), Conture and Kelly (1991) studied head and facial movements during the speech of a group of 30 stuttering and 30 nonstuttering children with a mean age of 54 months. They reported that the stuttering children had head-turns, blinks, and upper-lip raising significantly more often than nonstuttering children. Johnson and Associates (1959) asked parents of stuttering children and control parents whether their child had any "grimaces and odd body movements." Thirteen of 103 mothers (12.6 percent) of stuttering children responded "yes," but only one of 80 control mothers answered "yes." Two studies have asked parents whether their children's stuttering was associated with grimaces or body contortions at the time it began. Johnson and Associates (1959) reported that 23 of 149 (15.4 percent) mothers responded "yes" and Yairi (1983) reported that 4 of 22 parents (18.2 percent) responded "yes." Onslow, Harrison, and Jones (1993) asked whether grimaces occurred when stuttering first began, and 34 of 115 parents (29.6 percent) answered "yes."

There are three important recurring findings in the literature reviewed above. The first is that stuttering preschool children generally have far more disfluencies than nonstuttering preschool children, although it is certainly possible to find a nonstuttering child who has more disfluencies than a stuttering child. The second recurring finding is the prominence of part-word repetitions and prolongations in early stuttering. This has been replicated in many other studies not mentioned (for example, Bjerkan, 1980; Bloodstein & Grossman, 1981; Conture & Kelly, 1991; Culp, 1984; Yairi & Clifton, 1972; Westby, 1974). In particular, all this research conveys the impression that part-word repetitions (of sounds and syllables) are the most prominent of all disfluencies in early stuttering. That impression is bolstered considerably by some other studies which have used weaker methodologies than direct speech measures of children, but have been nonetheless remarkably consistent in their findings. These have been studies of parental recall of early disfluencies (Johnson & Associates, 1959; Onslow, Harrison, & Jones, 1993; Yairi, 1983) and studies of the type of disfluencies most likely to be judged as stuttering by listeners (Onslow, Gardner, Bryant, Stuckings, & Knight, 1992; Zebrowski & Conture, 1989). The impression is also confirmed by clinical descriptions of the development of the disorder presented by Van Riper (1971) and Bloodstein (1987).[1]

---

[1] There have been some single-subject case reports which suggest that final consonant repetitions might have been involved in stuttering onset. Mowrer (1987) studied the speech of a 2-year 10-month-old boy 3 weeks following the sudden onset of final-consonant repetitions which a parent thought was stuttering. Mowrer reported that during a 12 month period the boy showed a mean number of speech unit repetitions of 2.56 (range 1-7). Anecdotal reports by Rudmin (1984) and Camarata (1989) also suggest that final-consonant repetitions may be involved in stuttering onset, although the latter report makes no mention of stuttering. These reports are interesting because it is generally accepted that final-syllable repetitions are not typical of stuttering (Wingate, 1988).

The final recurring finding in all this literature is that part-word repetitions and prolongations are present in small proportions in the speech of nonstuttering preschool children. However, it is important to note that this does not mean that the part-word repetitions and prolongations of stuttering children are perceptually identical to those of nonstuttering children; just because two things can be described with the same term does not mean that they are essentially similar (Onslow, Gardner, Bryant, Stuckings, & Knight, 1992). For example, as noted previously, it is possible that the part-word repetitions of stuttering children will have more repetition units and be accompanied by head and facial movements. Further, it is worth reiterating the caution presented previously that disfluency categories need not be mutually exclusive. It is also worth noting that, in the literature mentioned above, observers have generally used only one term to describe each disfluency. It is entirely possible that the "part-word repetitions" of stuttering children are far more complex behaviors than those of nonstuttering children, and may in fact require several terms to describe them fully.

The following is a summary of results of studies of the speech of stuttering and nonstuttering preschool children:

1. Stuttering preschool-age children generally have more disfluencies than their nonstuttering counterparts.
2. Part-word repetitions of sounds and syllables and sound prolongations are common in stuttering preschool children. Part-word repetitions are probably the most distinctive feature of early stuttering.
3. Part-word repetitions and prolongations may occur in the speech of nonstuttering children, but it is not clear to what extent these resemble the part-word repetitions and prolongations of stuttering preschool children.
4. Stuttering preschool children may show more "clusters" of disfluencies when compared to nonstuttering children.
5. Stuttering children may have more repetition units in disfluencies than nonstuttering children, and they may have a greater range of repetition units per disfluency. However, at present the matter is open to question because there has been one report which found no differences.
6. Stuttering and nonstuttering preschool children may not be distinguishable by the durations of their disfluencies. However, this finding has yet to be replicated.
7. Early stuttering may involve head, face or body movements.

# Part Two:

# Bases of Behavioral Stuttering Management

# Introduction

## The nonbehavioral approach to stuttering management

Early in this century, Freud's ideas were a substantial influence on thinking about mental health. These conceptual developments were extensive and complicated, and it is not intended to review them here. However three of their salient features ought to be mentioned. First, disturbances to mental health were thought to have their origins in life history. Second, mental health disturbances were conceptualized with a medical model (Freud had a medical background), and so they were considered to be signs of an underlying disturbance. Finally, clinical management of mental health problems was directed to what was thought to be the underlying disturbance, not the signs of that disturbance.

In the first half of this century there were many descriptions of stuttering as a sign of underlying psychiatric problems, and many reports of stuttering being treated with psychoanalysis. Bloodstein (1987) outlines how moments of stuttering were explained in a symbolic fashion as a manifestation of repressed need. Explanations included stuttering as a reflection of "an infantile need for oral erotic gratification," "an attempt to satisfy anal erotic needs," "a covert expression of hostile or aggressive impulses that the person fears to express openly" or "the unconscious desire to suppress speech" (pp. 48-49). Bloodstein (1987) notes that it was theorized that children acquired such needs for stuttered speech in the same way that other "psychosexual fixations" are acquired:

> Broadly speaking, the fixations are thought to stem from early conflicts over the satisfaction of the special psychic needs of infancy—chiefly oral and anal eroticism, dependence, aggressiveness, and self-assertion. Such conflicts are generally considered to grow out of disturbed parent-child relationships and to be related to abnormal feeding or nursing behavior of the mother, excessively harsh or early weaning or toilet training, parental domination, overprotection or overanxiety, or other traumatic features of the family environment that frequently go back to the parents' own neurotic conflicts (pp. 59-60).

Lee Edward Travis formed the first academic speech-language pathology facility at the University of Iowa, and was influenced by the psychoanalytic approach to stuttering.[1] However, a different nonbehavioral view emerged from Iowa during the period 1930-1960 as Travis' students contemplated and researched the disorder. The essence of this view is that, in the first years of life, people who stutter acquire a belief that speech is difficult, and that belief persists into adulthood. It is that belief in the difficulty of speech, and apprehension about speech, which is responsible for the disorder. This view of stuttering and its management has been profoundly influential, particularly in management practices

---

[1] Johnson (1955) gives a background to origins of the speech pathology profession at the University of Iowa. Travis (1986) presents an interesting personal overview of his work, and provides an excellent insight into the psychoanalytic approach to stuttering treatment (Travis, 1971).

for young children, and it will be returned to at later stages. The features of the early nonbehavioral view of stuttering which emerged from the University of Iowa could be summarized as follows:

1.  The disorder is viewed as a manifestation of adverse cognitive and emotional factors.
2.  Management of the disorder involves attempts to rectify cognitive and emotional factors which are thought to be responsible for it.
3.  Direct elimination of stuttered speech is given little emphasis in the treatment process.

## The diagnosogenic theory

This theory is the best known manifestation of the nonbehavioral view of stuttering to emerge from the University of Iowa. Wendell Johnson's (1942) diagnosogenic theory was successful and extensively influential, and occupies an important place in the history of thought about the condition. It is dealt with more fully, and placed in perspective with regard to other theories, in a later section. In summary, the theory asserts that the cause of stuttering is its erroneous diagnosis by parents; in other words, they precipitate the development of stuttering by mistakenly believing that their child has begun to stutter. Johnson expressed this idea by saying that stuttering does not begin in the mouth of the child, but in the ear of the parent.

An important component of the diagnosogenic theory is that, at the time the diagnosis of stuttering is made by the parent, the child's speech is normal, consisting of the disfluencies that occur in the speech of all young children. Stuttering begins as the child attempts to avoid these normal disfluencies in response to parental pressure and expectations. In Johnson's view, the development of stuttering also is linked to unrealistic parental expectations and rigid child rearing practices. An interesting account of Johnson and his theory is provided by Bloodstein (1986), who was one of his students.

Johnson's diagnosogenic theory is no longer thought to be a satisfactory explanation of the etiology of stuttering (Bloodstein, 1986; 1987). Nonetheless, its influence on clinical practices from the 1940s has been extraordinary. The nature of that influence is well illustrated in Johnson's (1967) famous "open letter to the mother of a 'stuttering' child," which was widely distributed as information about the disorder:

> Do nothing at any time, by word or deed or posture or facial expression, that would serve to call Fred's attention to the interruptions in his speech. Above all, do nothing that would make him regard them as abnormal or unacceptable. (p. 550)

> Do not label or classify Fred as a "stutterer." If you do, you will have a very powerful tendency to treat him as if he were abnormal and unfortunate as the label suggests, and this may affect badly the way he feels about himself and weaken his self-confidence. (p. 551)

Apparently as a direct result of these ideas, the past three decades of clinical practice have been dominated by a concern that calling attention to early stuttering, or any other direct therapeutic effort, would hasten the development of the disorder. According to Wingate (1971), the influence of the theory extended even to the point where some clinicians were reluctant to acknowledge the presence of the disorder in their clients.

# The emergence of a behavioral approach to stuttering management

### Advanced stuttering

Ingham (1984) describes how the new doctrine of behaviorism, which emerged during the 1950s in clinical psychology, influenced thinking about stuttering. Ingham cites Kazdin's (1978) description of behaviorism as an approach concerned with present aspects, rather than historical aspects, of human problems, and "overt behavior change" as the primary way to determine the effectiveness of a treatment. The notion of "behavior" is integral to behaviorism. Johnson and Pennypacker (1980) offer the following definition:

> that portion of the organism's interaction with its environment that is characterized by detectable displacement in space through time of some part of the organism and that results in a measurable change in at least one aspect of the environment. (p. 48)

This definition excludes features of stuttering such as frustration and anxiety referred to in Part One, and includes only verbal and nonverbal features of stuttering such as blocks, prolongations, repetitions, grimaces, and so on. The 1960s saw the start of development of treatments for advanced stuttering that were designed specifically to *eliminate these and other stuttering behaviors*. These treatments, which gained widespread popularity, are based on prolonged speech (see page 22) and are discussed in detail in this text. Behavioral management practices such as prolonged speech are philosophically distinct from nonbehavioral approaches to stuttering management. One writing by proponents of nonbehavioral treatment illustrates the controversy surrounding the position that stuttering behavior is not a sign of an underlying problem but is the basic problem itself:

> The data that are produced by many of the behavioral suppressors are not recovery figures—they are suppression figures. The indecent scramble for ever and ever higher percentages, like 90 or 89 or 93, becomes totally meaningless. We suggest that the figures published on the establishment of fluency are mostly behavioral suppression figures and not ultimate recovery figures, and that the more successful the suppression, the less the chance of eventual recovery (Sheehan & Sheehan, 1984, p.150).

Siegel (1989) argues that there is value in a behavioral perspective on communication disorders. His argument is compelling if it is applied to the clinical management of stuttering: Regardless of what kind of disorder stuttering is, disordered behavior is at the interface of a person who stutters and that person's environment. In other words, even if stuttering is a sign of some underlying malaise, someone who stutters will still have disordered speech behaviors such as blocks or facial movements, or any of the observable features of the disorder described in Part One. As Andrews (1984b) notes, the disorder is not as private as many others, and everyone is aware that a person is affected by it because of its prominent problem behaviors. At the very least, then, a behavioral perspective on stuttering is relevant to clinicians, and elimination of the disruptive behaviors of the disorder will be a predominant part of clinical practice.

One asset that behaviorism can bring to stuttering management is accountability. The reason for this is that it incorporates "reliance upon basic research in psychology as a source of hypotheses about treatment and specific therapeutic techniques" (Kazdin, 1978, p. 35), rather than relying on unobservable, hypothetical processes thought to be responsible for human problems. More importantly, behaviors are observable, and therefore can be specified and measured. A combination of measurement and treatment is a powerful means to provide accountability in clinical practice by specifying treatment targets and determining whether those targets have been met. Another advantage to clinicians of appreciating the role of disordered behavior in stuttering is that there are various techniques—detailed in this text—which can control that disordered behavior to a clinically significant extent. If those techniques are used properly, then the problem speech behaviors which trouble clients can be rapidly eliminated or reduced.

Taken to an extreme, a behavioral approach to stuttering would overlook any internal, or unobservable, aspects of the disorder. However such an extreme viewpoint is in the interests of neither the client nor the clinician. Anxiety, frustration, and other feelings discussed in Part One may be a part of the disorder that clinicians will need to manage clinically. It also is the case that a range of nonbehavioral dimensions are critical in helping clients to eliminate stuttered speech; variables such as attitude to speaking, compliance, self-confidence and motivation.[1] To accept the importance of behavior in stuttering is not to reject the importance of those variables. It would be difficult to defend a treatment concerned only with the elimination of stuttered speech, and equally difficult to defend a treatment which paid no regard to the elimination of stuttered speech.

Baer (1988; 1989) has commented that it is important when managing a disorder to attend to what the client is complaining about. One possible error associated with a behavioral approach to stuttering is to assume that the client is, in fact, complaining about the problem speech behaviors of stuttering. On many—perhaps most—occasions that is what the client really is complaining about. Andrews (1984b) argues that stuttered speech is the most important client complaint in a clinic for stuttering treatment.[2] But it would be mismanagement if a client is given a behavioral treatment to eliminate stuttered speech when that client really did not complain about stuttered speech. What could clients be complaining about if not stuttered speech? One thing may be debilitating anxiety, or difficulty coping with the disorder, or perhaps the client may be complaining about having no support in attempting to live with stuttering. There is considerable clinical skill involved in determining exactly what the client's complaint is, but that skill needs to be acquired. If it is assumed, rather than established, that a client is complaining about disordered speech, then many inappropriate treatments may ensue.

Before leaving the discussion of the role of behaviorism in management of advanced stuttering, it is worth noting that there is no intrinsic reason why adults who stutter should eliminate stuttered speech. The condition is not medically harmful, and most people who have it are able to communicate with others. Many countries have legislation to prevent discrimination on the grounds of disability, so in those countries there are few occupations which are unavailable to people who stutter. It is the choice of the client whether stutter-free speech is a goal to be achieved. Many who stutter choose to live with the condition rather than attempt to eliminate or reduce stuttering. As with any long-standing problem behavior, the elimination of stuttered speech is a long-term undertaking, especially in the case of older clients. A fundamental task for a clinician is to help the client determine whether such an effort is justified.

## Early stuttering

The behavioral approach to early stuttering arrived decades later than with advanced stuttering. Perhaps one influence in that delay was the widespread—though overstated and misleading—belief that the majority of stuttering children do not require any intervention in

---

[1] These variables will be considered in Part Eight.

[2] Andrews (1984b) lists the following as other client complaints, in order of descending importance: "The handicap to communication produced by the stutter," "avoidance and reaction to speaking situations," and "negative attitudes to oneself as a speaker." (p. 243)

order for their stuttering to cease (see Part One). The enormously popular diagnosogenic theory (see above) certainly delayed the movement toward the elimination of early stuttered speech in young children: The first experimental attempt to draw young children's attention to their stuttering occurred in the early 1970s (Martin, Kuhl, & Haroldson, 1972), even though such experiments had been conducted on adult subjects since the 1950s.[1] But during the years in which behavioral treatments for advanced stuttering were developed, a daunting problem emerged which made it inevitable that a behavioral perspective on early stuttering would arrive. That problem was the difficulty in long-term elimination of stuttering behaviors in adults. It is clinical commonsense that more effective behavioral control of stuttering might be possible at the time when the disorder begins.

The first sign of an emerging consensus about this matter among clinicians occurred in a text based on a conference that dealt with management of stuttering in early childhood (Prins & Ingham, 1983). At that conference, clinicians from different backgrounds committed themselves to the notion of immediate and direct attention to stuttered speech. That consensus is one of the most important developments in the history of stuttering treatment:

> The belief remains intransigent that calling attention to disfluency in a young child may "cause" a problem of stuttering to emerge…in the face of even the clearest evidence that a child is having problems speaking fluently, our profession has, with a seemingly singular voice, given the advice to pay no attention—to ignore it. As an antidote, the contributors to this text have harmonized on a different note: when a young child shows persistent and unusual signs of disfluent speech… intervene—directly with the child and with the parents. (Prins & Ingham, 1983; p. 145)

# The focus of this text

This text reflects the influence of behaviorism in stuttering management in the following ways:

1. Treatments recommended are those designed to eliminate stuttered speech. Nonbehavioral aspects of stuttering are considered when they are directly pertinent to the elimination of stuttered speech. Management of nonbehavioral aspects of stuttering without reference to elimination of stuttered speech is beyond the scope of the text.
2. Speech measurement is emphasized as a means to provide accountability by prescribing treatment goals and by documenting progress toward and achievement of those goals.
3. Considerable value is placed on the public and verifiable nature of empirical research. Treatments are recommended only if their value has been demonstrated by the results of clinical and experimental research, or by theoretical perspectives that have been substantiated by research.

---

[1] Even though this experiment was successful, even today it is one of only a few of its kind. The Martin, Kuhl, & Haroldson experiment is considered in a later section.

# Speech Measures Used in Stuttering Management

## Functions of clinical measurement

### Accountability in clinical practice

One aspect of accountability is that the clinician should not be the only one who makes a judgement about the value of treatments. Their value also must be judged by various people and organizations. This is an important hallmark of modern professional clinical practice. One type of accountability is to clients or parents of clients, who have a right to information that will help them decide whether treatments are satisfactory. Another type of accountability is to the funding body that employs the clinician. This form of accountability can be politically valuable, especially in times where health care services are subject to budget restraints (Andrews, 1984b). Accountable clinical services can help speech pathology staff to demonstrate the value of their services to the community. Speech measures are an excellent contribution to clinical accountability, especially those that are direct indices of the presenting problem/s, and which can therefore be used to demonstrate how treatment eliminates those problems.

### Operation of treatments

Treatments for stuttering recommended in this text are, to varying extents, built around speech measures. This marriage of treatment and measurement methodology is a useful principle in the treatment of stuttering (Onslow & Ingham, 1987). The most direct example of this principle is programmed instruction (Mowrer, 1982), where speech measures are used to specify what the client must achieve during the treatment program in order to progress satisfactorily. Another example considered in this text is strategies to avoid post-treatment relapse which are built around measures of speech performance.

### Prescribing treatment goals

The clinician uses speech measures to make exact specifications of the goal of the treatment. The clinician also may prescribe a period of time during which treatment goals should be achieved. After this goal has been prescribed, the clinician and client, or the client's family, can determine at any time whether goals have been achieved or what progress has been made toward achieving them. This can assist all parties involved in treatment to determine whether treatment goals should be revised, or whether the treatment is worthwhile in terms of the amount of time involved.

### Treatment evaluation

It is fundamental for clinicians to know the effectiveness of the treatments they use so that clients and other clinicians can know what to expect of those treatments (Andrews, 1984b). Also, an ineffective treatment needs to be identified so that it can either be made effective or abandoned. Clinical research can only indicate, in a general sense, what treatments are likely to be effective. The work of determining whether a particular treatment is effective in a particular clinical setting must be done by clinicians. That work is referred to as program evaluation, and it assists clinicians in striving for constant improvements to their treatments. Without measures of speech performance, the work of evaluating the outcome of treatments and systematically improving them becomes impossible. Andrews (1984b) demonstrates the precision that speech measures can bring to describing the effectiveness of a treatment program:

> My average stutterer before treatment stutters on 12 percent of his syllables; immediately after the intensive phase of his treatment, he will stutter on 0.2 percent, and one and two years later he will stutter on about 2 percent of his syllables. (p. 242)

Andrews points out that this is far more informative and understandable than vague statements such as "most clients get better." Andrews also makes the point that, in a speech clinic, the cases who fail to achieve success are not as prominent as those who are successful; the unsuccessful cases return to the clinic frequently. Hence those unsuccessful cases may lead to a distorted impression of the effectiveness of a treatment.

## Client assessment

Speech measures obtained at the time of initial contact with the client can assist in assessing the severity and extent of the client's problem. In some cases they can assist in determining whether the client actually has a clinically significant problem. In order to do this, a variety of speech measures are necesary; it is unlikely that one speech measure obtained at initial assessment would be an adequate assessment of a client's problem. As considered in a later section, this is especially the case with children who are suspected of being in the early stages of stuttering.

## Facilitating client management responsibility

There is little chance a client will control stuttered speech if the client is dependent on the clinician for that control. This applies particularly after treatment gains have been established, and when the client attempts to remain free of stuttering for long periods of time. One way to promote clients' responsibility for their own treatment, or parents' responsibility for the treatment of their child, is to show them how to measure stuttering severity and related speech dimensions. The kinds of management responsibilities that can be assumed by clients through the use of speech measures include conducting treatment sessions at home, assessing everyday speech performance, and determining whether speech is satisfactory a long time after the conclusion of treatment.

## Communication with clients

Clinicians and clients need to communicate about the severity of the disorder and the progress of a treatment. Speech measures can provide a means for such communication. For example, at assessment the clinician can use various speech measures to inform the client how severe stuttering is in relation to other people who have the disorder. Another example of a clinician using speech measures to communicate with a client is when measures are made within the clinic at each visit. Those measures are useful in showing the client how much clinical progress is being made.

The clinician can benefit from the use of speech measures because they can provide information about the client's stuttering in everyday situations. As discussed in a later section, speech measures within the clinic are not likely to provide a full picture because stuttering is reactive to assessment and it may vary a great deal with speaking situations and time. So speech measures which the client obtains outside the clinic can inform the clinician precisely how severe stuttering has been since last contact. Such measures provide more information about how stuttering affects a client's life and whether the treatment is having any effect. With such knowledge the clinician is more likely to make appropriate management decisions and to be able to justify those decisions.

# Counts of speech events

The most commonly used speech measures involve counts of syllables spoken and syllables stuttered. They are sometimes called "objective" measures because it is thought that the presence of syllables or stutters can be recorded accurately and without observer bias. Unfortunately, the matter is not as straightforward as that, and is discussed in detail in Part Eight.

### Syllables or words spoken per minute (SPM or WPM)

This is a measure of speech rate which incorporates a count of the number of syllables or words spoken and the time taken to speak those syllables or words. The measure of time taken to speak the syllables or words does not include time when the client does not speak; when the client stops speaking, the timing stops. Here is an example of the calculation of syllables per minute (SPM):

> 1245 syllables spoken in 6.75 minutes
> SPM = 1245/6.75 = 184.4

A measure of speech rate is important in clinical practice because some treatment programs incorporate it within their procedures; those treatments involve systematic increases in speech rate. However, the real value of speech rate measures comes from the fact that speech rate has two relationships to stuttering severity. The first relationship is that stuttering may decrease when speech rate decreases (see page 23). Therefore, during some treatment procedures a measure of speech rate can provide a check that it is the treatment, not just the rate reduction, that reduces stuttering. The second clinically important relationship between speech rate and stuttering is an inverse one. In other words, if there is a lot of stuttering, then speech rate will tend to be low because stutters consume time. This means that speech rate measures can reflect the way that stutters consume time that otherwise would be occupied in producing speech. Because they reflect this aspect of the disorder, speech rate measures are a useful adjunct to stuttering severity measures. During a treatment program where a client's stuttering gradually improves, records of speech rate and stuttering measures almost always show an inverse relationship; as stuttering decreases, speech rate increases.

One limitation of SPM and WPM measures is that little is known about how fast any given person should speak, or about the range of speech rates during everyday speech. This is especially so in the case of children, for whom little more is known than that speech rate is a developmental variable.[1] For adults, some treatment programs give the impression that normal speech rate is around 200 SPM. However, there is such a wide range of normal speech rates that an average value has little meaning. It is also the case that speech rate may vary according to conversational partner. Another problem is that clinical attempts to time the intervals during which speech occurs have questionable accuracy. The only accurate way

---

[1] Data do exist for children's speech rates at different ages (for example, Amster 1984 as cited in Starkweather, 1987; Kowal, O'Connell, & Sabin, 1975; Peters & Guitar, 1991; Runyan & Runyan, 1993). However, these data were not gathered under identical conditions, so it is difficult for a clinician to use them as a guide to normal speech rates in children.

to measure the many brief pauses during speech is with a machine such as a waveform analyser or a sound spectrograph. It is also the case that speech rate measures do not necessarily reflect perceived speech rate. This means that if a client's SPM measures suggest slow speech (say 140 SPM) or fast speech (say 280 SPM) this does not necessarily mean that the client will be perceived as talking slow or fast.

With cases of early stuttering, there are some particular problems with measures of speech rate, because young children have shorter utterance lengths than adults. Many of the utterances of the youngest children who stutter will consist of one or two words. This makes it difficult to accurately time the duration of those utterances. It may be the case that there is no point in attempting measures of speech rate with preschool children, as was found in a study by Onslow, Costa, & Rue (1990).

## Percentage of syllables or words stuttered (%SS or %WS)

As discussed previously, the notion of a "moment of stuttering" is quite an important one. One reason is that it provides clinicians with a way to obtain an index of stuttering severity by counting the number of stutters that occur. Arguably this is the single most useful and common speech measure in stuttering treatment. In order to obtain %SS or %WS scores, the number of syllables or words are counted, along with the number of words or syllables that are stuttered. Normally, %SS or %WS scores are obtained at the same time as SPM or WPM scores, so the number of stutters can be shown as a percentage of the number of syllables or words spoken. Here is an example of the calculation of percent syllables stuttered:

1376 syllables spoken, 56 syllables stuttered
%SS = 56 /1376 x 100 = 4.1

One limitation of %SS and %WS measures is that they do not always reflect severity. Some clients will stutter quite infrequently, but each stutter will involve a long block. On the other hand, some clients stutter frequently, but each stutter is short and does not disrupt communication a great deal. As discussed above, a measure of speech rate may be able to offset this concern by reflecting the amount of time consumed by stuttering.

Measures based on syllables (%SS and SPM) seem to be favored more by clinicians than those based on words (%WS and WPM). One reason for this is that it is possible to stutter twice while saying a multisyllabic word. Clients who stutter severely will do this sometimes, and this will not be reflected in a %WS measure. Another reason is that many treatment programs are built around the syllable as a unit of speech. An additional consideration is that the number of syllables spoken per word may not be identical across speakers from different backgrounds, and it certainly differs between adults and young children. Another reason for preferring syllable-based measures is that it may have more face validity than word-based measures. As Wingate (1988) has argued, the problem of stuttering is "expressed at the level of the syllable" (p. 179). Stuttering is most likely to occur on a stressed syllable or on the first syllable of an utterance or a word. So, Wingate argues, syllabic factors are part of the expression of the disorder.

However, there is one advantage to word-based measures. Client or parent measures are important in clinical practice, and clients and parents are generally able to count words more easily than syllables. For the sake of convenience, syllable-based measures only will be referred to in the remainder of this text.

### Collecting %SS and SPM measures

Clinicians normally collect %SS and SPM measures concurrently. Syllables spoken are counted on-line, along with the number of spoken syllables that were stuttered. There are several audio and audio-visual training packages available to assist clinicians to learn to do this (for example, Burke, 1973; Ingham & Costello, 1987). Personal computer software packages, and stand-alone devices, are available for collecting %SS and SPM data. As the client speaks, the clinician presses a button for each nonstuttered syllable and another button for each stuttered syllable. These devices are sometimes referred to as "rating machines" or "disfluency counters." They have a built-in timer, which the clinician operates while conversing with the client and concurrently counting stutters and syllables.

Figure 1 shows a schematic record of a client's %SS and SPM scores over a period of time. Similar graphs of these and other speech measures are recorded in the client's file. As discussed previously, this presentation of speech measures assists in judging how well the client has progressed in treatment. Figure 1 also shows the common effect where SPM scores increase as %SS scores decrease.

FIGURE ONE: Weekly measures of %SS and SPM during the course of a client's treatment.

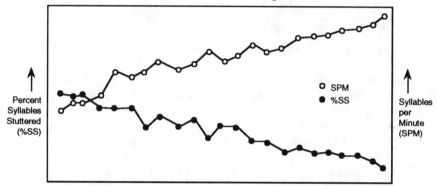

It is recommended that %SS measures are collected in real time at the start of each clinic visit. The start of each session is best because the treatment session itself is likely to cause a reduction in stuttering rate. Measuring %SS from a tape recording of the client's within-clinic conversation is not recommended because this is not a time-efficient procedure. Additionally, for clinicians who are learning skills in using the %SS measure, real-time rating is an important exercise. It is difficult to become proficient without real-time practice. There is more to real-time rating skills than accurate counting of syllables and stutters. The clinician needs to learn to simultaneously operate the device for counting syllables and stutters, conduct a conversation, and maintain eye contact with the client. This is a difficult set of skills to integrate with any client, but particularly so with preschool-age children. The reason is that, unlike adults, the clinician may have to work hard to engage a child in a conversation that resembles everyday speech. Such interactions with young children often require play activities and physical positions which restrict the clinician's use of equipment for counting syllables and stutters.

There are some special considerations for collecting %SS measures with preschool-age children. As with all speech measures involving young children, for the sake of validity it is best to converse with the child rather than prompt the child with stimulus materials such as story books. Some clinicians prefer to collect within-clinic %SS measures which are based on a conversation between the child and parent, because that is a more representative measure of everyday conversational speech. Certainly, this is an advisable procedure when a clinician first meets a young child. If this strategy is adopted, the clinician needs to arrange for a verbal interaction to occur between child and parent, and to rate such conversations on-line and unobtrusively. An audio or audiovisual monitoring system may be useful because it enables a covert assessment of child-parent conversation. Clinics with one-way observation windows are ideal for this purpose.

Compliance is another issue with obtaining %SS measures from young children. At the start of each session, adults will willingly converse with the clinician for the purpose of collecting this measure. However, young children may not be as compliant on all occasions. Considering all the things that have to be accomplished during a clinic session, it is difficult to justify allocation of more than 10 minutes to obtaining %SS measures. It is worth remembering that, with young children, the success of the session does not depend on collecting within-clinic data. Consequently, the procedure may be omitted on some occasions. This is preferable to either a parent or clinician wasting time trying to "drag" noninteractive utterances from a reluctant child. It is also worth remembering that the most important information about the child's speech comes from beyond the clinic, so it is not a significant problem if a within-clinic speech sample cannot be obtained, even at the initial clinical contact.

## Stutters per minute of speaking time (SMST)

The most useful speech measures for clinicians to use are %SS and SPM, but it is often not possible for clients/parents to learn how to collect them. Yet, for a number of reasons, it is crucial for clients/parents to collect beyond-clinic measures during their treatment. So on many occasions it is useful to teach the SMST measure to clients/parents in preference to %SS and SPM. The client/parent tape records conversational speech, and then at a later time the number of stuttering moments is counted and the accumulated speaking time is measured while listening to the tape recording. "Accumulated speaking time" refers to the amount of time during which the client speaks, with the timer turned off during periods when either the client pauses or another person speaks. No equipment is needed other than a cumulative stopwatch for measuring time, and a pen to count stuttering. Most clients/parents learn to count stuttering and measure speaking time concurrently. However, if necessary, the recording can be listened to twice, with stuttering counted at the first listening and time measured on the second listening. An advantage of SMST measures is that they are easier to obtain than %SS or SPM, and therefore are better suited for use by clients or their parents. One of their disadvantages is that they do not convey speech rate information. Below is an example how SMST is calculated:

> 12 stutters in 6.75 minutes accumulated speaking time
> $SMST = 12/6.75 = 1.78$

During the first few sessions of contact with a family, the clinician trains the client/parent to collect these data. Such training normally consists of the clinician listening to the tape together with the client/parent and providing instruction about what should be counted as a stutter. In addition, the clinician can have the client/parent practice stuttering identification using other speech samples which contain stuttering.

## Stutters per unit time (ST)

If SMST measures are unmanageable by clients/parents, ST measures may be collected instead. Although this procedure is not completely satisfactory, it is preferable to obtaining no beyond-clinic speech measures. This measure is useful when clients or parents fail to master the SMST measure. It is identical to SMST, except that the timing is not accumulated. In other words, the duration of the entire conversation is timed, including the time that the client was not speaking. For example, during breakfast a parent might use a wall clock to note a 10-minute period and count the child's stutters during that period. An advantage of

ST measures is that a stopwatch is not necessary and so they can be collected conveniently in real time without the need for tape recordings. Here is an example of calculation of ST:

15 stutters in a 10-minute period
ST = 15/10 = 1.50

Although this is the most convenient stutter-count speech measure for parents to collect, it is the least informative for the clinician. The reason is that it incorporates no measurement of the amount of speaking. This means that it is possible for two ST measures to be identical, but for much more stuttering to have occurred in one of the speech samples simply because there was more speech in that sample. Consequently, ST is a measurement procedure that should be avoided unless the client/parent cannot manage any other technique.

In some cases where parents or clients fail to learn ST measures, the clinician may opt to collect beyond-clinic speech data. One way of doing this is for the clinician to telephone the child or client at home once or twice per week and rate speech on-line for %SS and SPM during conversation. Another option is for the client/parent to present tape recordings to the clinician each week for rating. Although both these alternatives are inconvenient for the clinician, it is the only recourse available in some rare cases. It is difficult to imagine that accountable management of a client could occur without the clinician having access to some beyond-clinic measures based on stutter counts.

## Additional speech-event measures for assessment

The measures described above are designed for use during day-to-day clinical practice. However, additional measures are available for use when the clinician requires a detailed description of the client's stuttering, such as during an initial assessment. To obtain these measures it is necessary to tape record the client. The procedures below are based on suggestions made by Costello and Ingham (1984a) and Starkweather, Gottwald, and Halfond (1990).

*Mean duration of stutters* can be calculated by tape recording a speech sample and timing the duration of 10 randomly-selected stutters. The total duration of these stutters is then divided by 10 to calculate mean stuttering duration. *Duration of the three longest stutters;* while the client is speaking and being tape recorded, the clinician can note the tape counter value at the place where the longest stutters occur. This makes it quicker to scan the tape recording later to find the three longest stutters. *Percent-time disfluency* is described by Starkweather, Gottwald, and Halfond (1990). It indicates the portion of the child's speaking time spent in stuttered speech. A stopwatch is used to measure the duration of stutters in the speech sample. *Mean number of repetitions* pertains to whole- and part-word repetitions. The number of repetitions is counted for 10 randomly-selected stutters which involve repetition of this kind, and the mean is calculated (for example, mu-mu-mu-mummy is three repetitions). *Number of the three longest repetitions* can be obtained in a manner similar to "duration of the three longest stutters" above. The clinician reports the number of repetitions involved in the three longest repetitions. *Mean duration of stutter-free intervals* can be calculated from the tape recording by measuring the duration of 10 randomly-selected stutter-free intervals, and dividing this total duration by 10. Duration of stutter-free intervals can be measured using seconds or syllables spoken. *Duration of the three longest stutter-free intervals* may be obtained in a manner similar to "duration of the three longest stutters" above.

The following is an example of how a clinician might describe a client's stuttering using the speech measures presented in the above sections. Note that the clinician reports the number of syllables and the speaking time involved in the measures.

In a 3,000-syllable conversation (accumulated speaking time 14.2 minutes) stuttering occurred at a rate of 3.9 %SS, with a speech rate of 211.3 SPM (equipment set to manual timing). Stutters were blocks, prolongations or part-word repetitions. During some blocks, mouth opening and tongue protrusion occurred, which was accompanied by blinking. Prolongations were often accompanied by a slight forward head thrust. The mean duration of stutters was 1.6 seconds, and the three longest stutters noted in this sample were 23.8 seconds, 16.8 seconds, and 4.2 seconds. The mean duration of stutter-free intervals in the sample was 24.9 syllables, and the duration of the three longest stutter-free intervals were 97 syllables, 82 syllables, and 73 syllables.

# Rating-scale speech measures

These measures do not involve the counting of speech events. Instead, an observer uses an ordinal scale to assign a value to some speech dimension. This means that measures obtained in this way are based on the perception of observers. A common misconception is that rating scale measures are of less value than measures based on speech event counts because they are "subjective." However, at least from a clinical viewpoint, such a view is questionable. Arguably what determines whether a clinical measure is useful is its convenience, its reliability and its validity. The convenience of rating scales is obvious; they involve no equipment and they are effortless to administer. They are also valid because they are based on the perception of observers, which is obviously relevant in determining the severity of a communication disorder.

### Speech naturalness

Prolonged-speech treatments for stuttering (see page 22) require the client to use a novel way of speaking. As will be discussed in Part Six, one side-effect of this is that, although speech may be stutter-free, it does not sound natural. Martin, Haroldson, and Triden (1984) and Martin and Haroldson (1992) developed a 9-point scale which can be used by clinicians to measure the dimension of speech naturalness, as follows:

> 1 = highly natural
> 9 = highly unnatural

There is some research which shows that this scale is valid because it can distinguish between the speech of people who do not stutter and people who have been treated for stuttering (Ingham, Gow, & Costello, 1985; Metz, Schiavetti & Sacco, 1990; Onslow, Hayes, Hutchins, & Newman, 1992). Some studies have also shown how the scale can be useful in treatment because clinicians can use it to *feed back* speech naturalness scores to clients to help them to achieve natural-sounding speech (Ingham, Ingham, Onslow, & Finn, 1989; Ingham, Martin, Haroldson, Onslow, & Leney, 1985; Ingham & Onslow, 1985). How this can be done will be described in Part Four. Speech naturalness ratings are normally based on either 15-second, 30-second or 60-second intervals of speech.[1]

### Stuttering severity

A scale of stuttering severity is an extremely useful clinical tool. Informally, clinicians often refer to clients' stuttering as "mild," "moderate," or "severe." Sometimes a five-category system is used by adding the terms "mild-moderate" and "moderate-severe." These categories are usually determined simply according to the judgment of the clinician when

---

[1] There is personal computer software available to assist clinicians to gather speech naturalness scores on-line (Fowler & Ingham, 1986).

listening to the client speaking. However, there is available a scoring system which is designed to assist clinicians in determining a severity category into which a client falls. This system is referred to as the Stuttering Severity Instrument (SSI) (Riley, 1972) and is used by many clinicians and researchers. The following 10-point scale of stuttering severity was researched by Eve, Onslow, Andrews, and Adams (1993):

> 1 = normal speech
> 10 = extremely severe stuttering,

Clinicians may find severity rating scales useful for managing any client, but they are a particularly useful complement to %SS and SPM measures with preschool-age children. The procedure does not depend on instrumentation which might disrupt verbal interaction with very young children. More importantly, the child does not need to comply with the measurement procedure, and need not even be aware that it is occurring. This covert nature of severity scaling makes it a convenient and valid assessment tool for young children. Further, the scale allows measures to be made more frequently than is convenient with stuttering-count procedures, and in situations that would not be practical for stuttering-count measures. This is a particularly important advantage of severity scaling because, as discussed in Part One, early stuttering can show large variations in severity from day to day and even from situation to situation. Clinicians stand to benefit from a such a convenient method for parents to supply constant information about the severity of their children's stuttering.

Some time shortly after the initial contact with the parents of a preschool child, the clinician assists them in making a list of from five to ten speaking situations which can easily be contrived or which occur regularly during the child's life. An example of a contrived speaking situation for the purposes of severity rating is a phone call to a relative, and examples of routinely-occurring speaking situations are bath times, meal times, in the car on the way to preschool, talking on the telephone, playing with a parent in the garden, and bedtime. Situations can be chosen also to represent when the child is most likely to stutter. Severity ratings are made by parents each day, or each other day. Each day (or each other day) a parent selects one of the speaking situations from the list, and listens for 5 minutes while their child speaks in that situation. At the end of the 5-minute interval, the parent assigns a severity rating and records it. It is useful if parents graph severity ratings so that they and clinicians can easily inspect trends in severity scores over a period of time. A variation on this procedure which may be useful on some occasions is for parents to assign a severity rating each evening, and to base that rating on the child's speech during the entire day, rather than on a selected 5-minute interval.

Useful as severity scaling is, it is important to recognize its limitations. One limitation is that it does not provide information about the number of stutters in a child's speech. Nonetheless, in a clinical setting such a shortcoming may not be too serious if a severity scale can rank order speech samples in the same fashion as %SS scores. The report by Onslow, Andrews and Costa (1990) suggests that this might be the case with some clients.

Although it is useful to collect daily speech assessments of a young child, it is important to avoid placing excessive demands on a family in making such assessments. It can hinder effective management if a clinician obtains a commitment from parents to collect daily severity measures, and those parents become stressed in honoring that commitment. On some occasions, the clinician might choose to modify the procedure so that severity scale scores are obtained by the parent on each second day. Generally, though, if severity rating situations are chosen which are part of everyday life the technique intrudes little into family routine.

There has been considerable research on the use of severity scales to measure stuttered speech. However, much of that research has been directed to short speech samples, with little attention paid to severity ratings of intervals of speech which would normally be used for clinic assessment, such as 5 or 10 minutes. There are some data, though, which indicate that listeners might be able to use a rating scale to reliably and validly measure stuttering severity in speech samples ranging from 1 to 5 minutes duration (Cullinan & Prather, 1968; Eve, Onslow, Andrews, & Adams, 1993; Martin & Haroldson, 1992; Onslow, Andrews, & Costa, 1990).

## Determining the reliability and validity of beyond-clinic measures

Because speech measures outside the clinic are so important to the treatment process, it is crucial that the clinician carefully monitors the reliability and validity of those measures. Otherwise poor management decisions may be made because of faulty information about the child's progress in treatment.

The most fundamental requirement for a useful speech measure is intrajudge reliability (sometimes referred to as "consistency"). If a person does not produce similar scores for the same speech sample on two different occasions, then speech measures collected by that person may be of limited value. Client/parent intrajudge reliability for SMST and severity scores can be assessed by retaining the recordings on which the first two SMST scores are based. The clinician can have the client/parent also assign a severity score to those recordings, and then place them aside for a week. After a week, the recordings can be given back to the client/parent for re-measurement of SMST and severity. For severity scores, an acceptable margin is a difference of plus or minus one scale value between the parent's first and second score. For SMST scores, a recommended acceptable margin is a difference of less than 10 percent between the parent's first and second score.

Interjudge reliability is the extent to which different people's scores agree. Interjudge reliability of severity scores between clinician and parent can be assessed by comparing a parent severity rating with a clinician severity rating at each clinic session. This can be done by asking the parent to assign a severity rating to the child's speech just after the clinician has collected within-clinic %SS measures at each clinic visit. The clinician asks the parent to assign a severity score to the child's speech that was just rated. This procedure enables the clinician to check that the parent is not assigning unrealistic severity ratings to a child's speech. On occasions, it will be necessary to discuss appropriate severity ratings with parents.

The validity of a speech measure can be determined by comparing it to another measure. The validity of SMST and severity scores can be assessed by inspecting a graph where both measures are displayed. If the two measures depict the same trends in the client's stuttering over a period of time, as occurs in Figure 3 on page 84, then they are valid measures of the client's stuttering severity. A more direct way to assess the validity of SMST and severity scores is to arrange for one or both the SMST recordings each week to be collected in one of the speaking situations used for obtaining severity scores (see above). For example, one SMST measure each week can be based on a recording of the child in the car, and that conversation can also be one of those the parent attends to each day for 5 minutes and assigns a severity score. Then, if changes in the SMST score and the severity score for that situation are not reflected in both measures, the clinician knows that there is something wrong with the validity of one or both the measures.

# Graphing speech measures during treatment

It is recommended that the within- and beyond-clinic measures outlined above are recorded graphically to facilitate communication with parents and facilitate inspection of data trends. Speech measures can be added at each clinic visit. Figure 3 on page 84 shows an example of how a clinician might record speech measures in a client's file. That example is for a preschool-age client, and it shows a straightforward example of steady improvement over a number of weeks. However, many other trends may appear which are extremely useful for the clinician to know about. For example, an initial improvement trend might stabilize, with no further change after several weeks of treatment. In management of early stuttering, this can indicate to the clinician that parents may have ceased to conduct the treatment sessions with the same diligence as at the start of the treatment. Alternatively, it may mean that the way the treatment is being conducted is no longer appropriate. Another example of a clinically important trend with early stuttering is cyclical variation in severity, which can occur during treatment because it is one characteristic of the early stages of the disorder (see pages 66-67). Graphical depictions of this trend are important in determining whether treatment is effective or whether the child has improved merely as a part of that cycle of severity.

# Conditions that may bias speech measures

## Speaking situations

Many people who stutter tell clinicians that certain situations in their lives are consistently associated with more, or less, stuttering.[1] A person's stuttering may be more severe in front of a large audience, and less severe when speaking to one or two people. This isn't surprising, considering that most people find it unsettling to speak to a group of people if they are not accustomed to doing so. It also appears that certain attributes of the person being spoken to can influence stuttering severity, so that less stuttering might occur with a "friendly" conversationalist than with a formal and authoritative figure. For example, someone who stutters might not stutter much in conversation with a spouse, but might stutter a lot when talking to a person in authority at work.

Clients often report that situations with pressures to produce speech in a short time are troublesome. Examples of such situations are being asked to place an order in a restaurant or asking for a train ticket. In the case of children, probably the most common pressure situation is speaking during class or—even worse—in front of a class. A speaking situation which adult clients perceive to be notoriously difficult is the telephone (Leith & Timmons, 1983). It is worth noting that a client's perception that a speaking situation is difficult does not necessarily mean that the client stutters more that situation; a situation may be perceived as difficult because it makes the speaker feel uncomfortable.

These effects may bias clinical speech measures, which can result in misleading information about a client's stuttering severity. For example, %SS scores collected while a client is at home speaking to a spouse may not provide a realistic assessment of the extent of the stuttering problem. In the interests of a complete assessment of a client's stuttering, it is useful to measure speech under conditions which may increase stuttering. For example, a client could be required to speak to a stranger, speak on the telephone, or speak to a group

---

[1] In contrast, many people who stutter tell clinicians that they cannot predict when speech difficulties will occur, and that unpredictability is one of the worst things about the condition.

of people. Speech is assessed in such situations as a routine part of many adult treatment programs outlined in later sections. For example, clients may be required to address a group, speak on talk-back radio, or speak to shopkeepers.

## The act of measurement

Stuttering is one of many human problems that may be responsive to the act of overt assessment. For example, a chain smoker whose spouse is counting the number of cigarettes smoked is less likely to smoke when the spouse is not present. This can be the case with stuttering; it may decrease when it is being measured simply because the client does not want to be observed stuttering. Stuttering may also decrease under measurement conditions because of discriminated learning. This refers to when the client learns to be stutter free only in the presence of certain stimuli (referred to as discriminative stimuli), such as a clinician, a treatment setting, or a treatment instrument . It is a common problem in the management of some clients that stuttering disappears in the presence of such stimuli, but reappears when those stimuli are no longer present. This effect can be so dramatic that someone who is stuttering severely in everyday life can become completely stutter-free in the presence of a clinician who is monitoring or measuring stuttering.[1]

The clinical relevance of this is considerable. Indications of stuttering severity obtained from overt measurements—especially measurements made in a speech clinic—may be biased and lead to misinformation about a client's stuttering severity. Another aspect of reactivity to measurement is that it can be frustrating, to both the client and the clinician, if stutter-free speech is present only when speech is being monitored or measured by a clinician. One of the worst things a clinician can hear is "there is no problem here in the clinic, but stuttering happens all the time at home."

The effects of bias caused by the act of assessment can be offset by covert measurement. This is measurement of the client's speech by the clinician, parent or spouse without the client's knowledge. This procedure can be unethical if not handled correctly, and it should not occur without the prior agreement of the client. Before treatment begins, the clinician can obtain the client's approval for the procedure. If it is explained why covert assessment may be necessary, few clients object. Of course, covert assessment is pointless if the client becomes aware of the procedure, so the success of such assessment depends on the clinician's ingenuity and creativity. One approach is for a clinician who is unknown to the client to telephone the client on a fabricated pretext, such as a telephone survey. Another approach is to have a relative or spouse occasionally make surreptitious tape recordings of the client, or to surreptitiously collect a speech measure such as ST (see page 40) on-line as the client speaks.

---

[1] If a client has had intensive treatment where a clinician has used a machine for counting syllables and stutterings on-line (see pages 38-39), the mere sight of that machine after the treatment program may produce stutter-free speech.

# Eliminating Stuttered Speech: Some Critical Concepts

The most fundamental skill in eliminating stuttered speech is to understand basic concepts about how to do it. Those concepts guide all the procedures used in clinical practice. Reliance on clinical procedures rather than the concepts that underlie them can lead to inflexible management practices which will not provide optimal benefits for clients. This idea recurs throughout this text. Parts Three and Four describe various procedures that clinicians and researchers recommend for eliminating stuttered speech. In some cases, those procedures, exactly as they are recommended, will be suitable for an individual client. But in most cases they will not. Most times, clinical practice conducted as a set of predetermined procedures does not give clients the best possible assistance to eliminate their stuttering. The best help clients can get comes from a clinician who (1) understands concepts of how to eliminate stuttered speech (2) is prepared to use those concepts flexibly and creatively to formulate clinical procedures.

Before proceeding, though, the meaning of the phrases "eliminating stuttered speech" and "stutter-free speech" as used in this text need some clarification. Strictly speaking, many treatments that clinicians and clients consider successful do not completely "eliminate" stuttering or produce speech which is completely "stutter-free." So, although expressions such as "nearly eliminate" and "virtually stutter-free" might be more correct on some occasions, they are not used here for the sake of convenience.

## Prolonged speech

As discussed in Part One, there are many speaking conditions which can control stuttering. Treatment reports by Goldiamond (1965) prompted modern interest in the use of a particular way of speaking based on the effects of DAF. In effect, DAF prompts a speaker to use a novel speech pattern, which Goldiamond termed "prolonged speech." Goldiamond devised procedures to shape this unnatural speech pattern towards natural sounding speech. Currently there are many speech patterns derived from this procedure which are used in the treatment of stuttering, but the technique is referred to generically as "prolonged speech."

Prolonged speech has one distinguishing feature which qualifies it as a behavioral treatment: It replaces the problem behaviors of stuttering with speech behaviors that are incompatible with stuttering. In other words, stuttered speech is replaced with prolonged speech. This is a common component of management of problem behaviors. For example, someone may replace the smoking of a cigarette with the eating of an apple, or replace drinking alcohol with the drinking of a non-alcoholic beverage. Clearly, though, implementing such an idea with a problem behavior might be more difficult in practice than it sounds in theory. This certainly is the case when the idea is applied to stuttering treatment.

Prolonged speech treatments for stuttering are not straightforward, and they are not an ideal solution to the problem of stuttering. This is because they require the client to make a permanent change to customary speech. They require many hours to complete, and they involve numerous problems which are considered in later sections of the course. The most troublesome of these problems is that prolonged speech may result in speech that sounds unnatural to listeners, which feels unnatural to clients, and which may require unusual attention to the act of speaking. These negative features are balanced by the advantage that some clients may be able to use prolonged speech to control the effects of their condition on daily life.

# Response contingent stimulation (operant methodology)

Some human problems can be viewed as "operants." According to Costello and Ingham (1984b), this term describes

> those responses, or classes of responses, that are controlled (changed in frequency or form) by their consequences, that is, by environmental events that follow their occurrence. (p. 187-188)

Another feature of an operant is that it is created and controlled by such environmental events. This is certainly not the case with stuttering, but it certainly shows "operant-like" properties to the extent that it can be *controlled* by environmental consequences. Those consequences are referred to as stimuli, and if they occur soon after the appearance of a stutter (or after a period of stutter-free speech), then they are referred to as response contingent stimuli (RCS).

FIGURE TWO: Stimulus and contingency arrangements associated with reinforcement and punishment (adapted from Costello and Ingham, 1984). The arrows depict either the increase or decrease of behaviors.

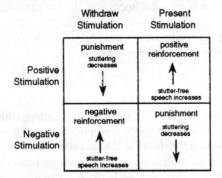

There are many kinds of RCS and many ways of presenting them. *Reinforcement* refers to when contingent stimulation *increases* the rate at which a behavior occurs. There are two types of reinforcement. The first type is negative reinforcement, which is the removal of a negative stimulus contingent on the occurrence of a behavior. The second type is positive reinforcement, which is the presentation of a positive stimulus contingent on the occurrence of a behavior. *Punishment* refers to when contingent stimulation *decreases* the rate at which a behavior occurs. There are two kinds of punishment. The first type is removal of a positive stimulus contingent on the occurrence of a behavior, and the second type is the presentation of a negative stimulus contingent on the occurrence of a behavior.[1] Figure 2 presents punishment and reinforcement schematically. Reducing or increasing behaviors with RCS is

---

[1] Terms "reinforcement" and "punishment" do not refer to a stimulus, but to the effect of the stimulus on the response rate in question. In this correct sense of the terms, reinforcement has not occurred unless a behavior has increased its rate of occurrence, and punishment has not occurred unless a behavior has decreased its rate of occurrence.

called operant conditioning, and the various ways of doing this are known collectively as *operant methodology*.

Operant methodology is used in the treatment of stuttering by punishing stuttering and reinforcing periods of stutter-free speech. Many kinds of verbal and tangible stimulation are used in treatment procedures outlined in this text.

# Programmed instruction

Much of the elimination of stuttering consists of the teaching of new behaviors to clients or the prompting and reinforcing of existing behaviors. Programmed instruction is one way that clinicians can accomplish these tasks. The benefits of programmed instruction in teaching are well known, and this procedure is a fundamental part of clinical practice with communication disorders (Costello, 1977; Mowrer, 1982). It has an important place in many treatments for stuttering. The principles of shaping enable the client to achieve successive approximations to the treatment target of stutter-free speech. In this process, speech performance criteria for the client change systematically. The progress of the client through the treatment program depends on achieving those criteria.

One of the most popular formats for programmed instruction described later in this text is prolonged speech treatment in an intensive setting. In this format, programmed instruction is used to replace stuttered speech with an unnatural sounding speech pattern, and then is used to shape that speech pattern toward more natural sounding speech. Subsequently, programmed instruction is used to assist the client to acquire the skill of using that new speech pattern in everyday speaking situations. The client is assigned treatment tasks of producing stutter-free speech in easy speaking situations, such as talking to a friend or a clinician, and then more difficult tasks are prescribed, such as talking to a stranger or in front of a group.

Other popular programmed instruction procedures considered in this text are based on the Extended Length of Utterance (ELU) program (Costello, 1983). The client is required initially to produce a single, stutter-free syllable, and then is required to produce two, three, four, and so on, stutter-free syllables. Eventually the client is required to produce 30 seconds, 60 seconds, and eventually 5 minutes of stutter-free speech. The ELU program does not incorporate prolonged speech, although the clinician has the option to do this.

# Nonprogrammed instruction

Nonprogrammed instruction is a less formal and structured way of assisting someone to produce a desirable behavior. Consider a child who does not say "thank you" when given something by an adult. Most adults think that their children should display this desirable behavior, and nonprogrammed instruction is one way they might teach a child to do this. In a nonsystematic manner, the child can be prompted to say "thank you" from time to time, and praised from time to time for saying "thank you," and occasionally corrected for failing to do so. Contrast this with a programmed approach to the matter. The child could be given a treatment target of saying "thank you" at appropriate times on four successive occasions, and given a formal reward for reaching that criterion. Then, the next task could be to say "thank you" at appropriate times on five successive occasions, and so on. Of course this example is for the purpose of illustration only, because there would never be any need to go to the trouble of programmed instruction to teach a child to say "thank you" in a socially acceptable way. However, there is often a need in communication disorders to take the trouble to use programmed  instruction. An important clinical decision in the treatment of stuttering is whether or not programmed instruction is a necessary part of a management strategy.

Programmed instruction has always been prominent in stuttering management, because it was incorporated within Goldiamond's (1965) prolonged speech procedure which was mentioned above, and this technique became popular throughout the world. However, as will be discussed in Part Four, programmed instruction may not be necessary or desirable with many clients who need to be treated with prolonged speech. Now that clinicians treat cases of early stuttering, nonprogrammed instruction is a more common part of the clinician's repertoire. Two- and three-year old children are not amenable to the formality and structure associated with programmed instruction. Nonprogrammed instruction is also suitable for use with cases of early stuttering because, as considered previously, such cases probably do not involve a skill deficit and hence are likely to respond to treatments aimed at prompting and reinforcing the appearance of stutter-free speech.

# Treatment Targets in Eliminating Stuttered Speech

## Stutter-free speech

Stutter-free speech can be targeted in two ways. There are treatments which focus on eliminating stuttering, and there are treatments which focus on increasing the duration of speech intervals which do not contain stuttering. Some treatments focus on both these targets simultaneously. As a general rule, treatments for children need to focus on stutter-free speech far more than they focus on stuttering. The reason for this is that it creates a positive emphasis to the treatment, which is important in promoting behavior change in children.

## Self monitoring

If clients are to eliminate stuttered speech, then they should know when they are stuttering. It is difficult to imagine that any client would be able to succeed in a treatment program if that client was not aware when stuttering occurred. Consequently, clinicians often prescribe for clients a variety of tasks designed to train them in monitoring for the occurrence of stuttered speech. One example would be the use of a small hand-held counter which a client would use to count stutters as they occurred. An additional benefit of self monitoring is that, in effect, the procedure is RCS and hence it may contribute to the control of stuttering. In treatment of preschool-age children, monitoring for stuttered speech is a treatment target, and parents reward their children for accurate self monitoring.

## Self evaluation

Self evaluation means something similar to self monitoring, but with an important difference. In self monitoring the client merely invigilates and, perhaps, records the occurrence of stuttering. But with self evaluation the client assesses performance. This is an indispensable part of any treatment program because it encourages clients to be responsible for managing their stuttering. Again, in the case of preschool-age clients, correct self evaluation is a treatment target that parents reward.

## Compliance

Treatment will not work unless the client cooperates fully with it, and treatments may fail because the client does not cooperate. Compliance itself can be used as a treatment goal. In other words, in cases where it is appropriate, the client can be trained to comply with treatment requirements. For example, consider an initial treatment session where an adult client had been trained in the first steps in a treatment program. The clinician might then ask the client to practice those steps on three nights during the next week, tape record those practice sessions, and mail the recording to the clinician. The clinician could tell the client that on receipt of the recordings, a second training session would be scheduled. What is occurring here is that the clinician is attempting to reinforce compliance.[1] In the case of young children—for stuttering or any other speech disorder—reinforcement of compliance is an essential part of clinical procedures.

## Generalization

The terms "establishment" or "instatement" refer to the stage of treatment when the client has achieved the target level of stutter-free speech. However, that is by no means the most important part of stuttering treatment. After having acquired stutter-free speech, the client must generalize that gain. Stokes and Baer (1977) define "generalization" as the appearance of the required behavior/s in various nontreatment conditions without the training that occurred during treatment. The nontreatment conditions referred to by Stokes and Baer include different people and different settings. Generalization also may be said to have occurred when only a limited part of the training is required for the appearance of the target behavior in nontraining conditions. In short, generalization may be claimed when treatment conditions no longer support, or they provide less support for, behavior change. In the case of stuttering treatment, generalization is when the client shows signs of stutter-free speech in everyday speaking situations when there is no sign of anything connected with treatment which might be responsible for this.

## Maintenance

Maintenance can be thought of as a special case of generalization; the appearance of the target behavior in non-training conditions *over time* , in addition to across people and settings. In stuttering treatment, clinicians seem generally to agree that at least several years is the period of time during which clinical gains need to be maintained for a treatment to be considered successful. The term "relapse" is used to describe a situation where an attempt to maintain treatment benefits has been unsuccessful and the client has returned to stuttered speech. These last two treatment goals of generalization and maintenance are so critical that they are considered separately in the following sections.

---

[1] Using compliance as a clinical goal often reveals that the client is not prepared to undertake a behavioral treatment for stuttering, which is invaluable information in helping that client with the problem of stuttering. With the example given here, the client may fail on three separate occasions to mail the tape of the practice sessions, in which case the clinician would begin to explore the reasons for that noncompliance.

# Generalization and Maintenance in Eliminating Stuttered Speech

There are several reasons why generalization and maintenance are considered together in this section. This first is that, as indicated above, they are much the same thing, with maintenance being a special case of generalization. Because this is the case, many of the procedures known to promote generalization may also promote maintenance, and so the topics can be discussed at the same time. Another reason to consider generalization and maintenance together is that *these two notions constitute a definition of successful treatment.* Stuttering cannot be considered to be controlled unless it improves in everyday speaking situations for a substantial period of time. Or, if the client specifies that stutter-free speech is required in only one or a few speaking situations, a claim of success depends on the achievement of stutter-free speech in that situation/s.

## Clinical procedures to promote generalization and maintenance

Stokes and Baer (1977) reviewed procedures for generalization of behavior change, and Ingham and Onslow (1987) described the use of those procedures in stuttering treatments. Little is known empirically about what will improve generalization in stuttering treatments, especially in the case of children. However, the Stokes and Baer procedures are a valuable commonsense approach to the issue. The section headings below are from Stokes and Baer (1977).

### Sequential modification

This is a programmed instruction procedure where the client progressively demonstrates mastery of treatment targets in a sequence of speaking situations that have been arranged by the client and/or parent into a hierarchy of difficulty. The idea is that this will facilitate generalization of stutter-free speech. Sequential modification is a fundamental component of the intensive prolonged speech treatments referred to on page 22. In these treatments, when stutter-free speech has been achieved the client completes a sequence of tape-recorded speaking assignments in situations outside the clinic. These are arranged in a hierarchy from the least to the most difficult. This part of the treatment is sometimes referred to as "transfer." "Transfer" is sometimes used as a synonym for "generalization," but this is not strictly correct because the former term refers only to one of many specific techniques for promoting generalization.

With preschool-age children, there seems not to be the need for the formal programming with sequential modification that there might be for older clients, and it is rare for clinicians to use this technique with this age group. However the technique may be required with older children. In the case of children who cannot operate hand-held tape recorders, the parent may be able to tape record the speaking assignment. Alternatively, the parent might conduct sequential modification by monitoring for stuttering on-line as the child attempts the various speaking situations. However, most children who are old enough to require sequential modification as part of their treatment can learn to use a cassette recorder correctly.[1]

TABLE ONE: A general form of a sequential modification program to achieve generalization, adapted from Ingham (1987). See text for explanation.

| Step | Assignment | Criteria for Pass | Pass: Go To | Fail: Go To |
|------|-----------|-------------------|-------------|-------------|
| S1   | a         | See text          | S1b         | S1a         |
|      | b         |                   | S1c         | S1a         |
|      | c         |                   | .           | .           |
|      | d         |                   | .           | .           |
|      | e         |                   | S1f         |             |
|      | f         |                   | S2a         | S1a         |
| .    | .         |                   | .           | .           |
| .    |           |                   |             |             |
| .    | .         |                   | .           | .           |
| S6   | a         |                   | S6b         | S6a         |
|      | b         |                   | S6c         | S6a         |
|      | c         |                   | .           | .           |
|      | d         |                   | .           | .           |
|      | e         |                   | S6f         | .           |
|      | f         |                   | Maintenance | S6a         |

Table 1 shows the general structure of a performance-contingent sequential modification generalization procedure, based on that devised by Ingham (1987). The steps S1-S6 represent a number of speaking situations that have been ordered in a sequence from least to most difficult. Each step contains six assignments. Criteria for passing assignments are a prescribed number of syllables that must be tape recorded during a conversation, and less than a certain percentage of syllables stuttered. As an example of specific performance requirements of a sequential modification program, Ingham (1987) prescribes six steps each consisting of six speaking assignments of 1,300 syllables duration. Criteria for passing assignments are speech which contains zero stuttering and which also conforms to a criterion of speech naturalness (see page 42) which is formulated individually for each client. The performance contingent nature of the program is shown in the last two columns of Table 1. When the client has progressed through the sequential modification program, the clinician may decide that the client should begin the Maintenance Phase or may decide that further generalization training is necessary.

---

[1] Lapel microphones are useful because they facilitate a clear recording of speech .

## Introduce to natural maintaining contingencies

This approach to generalization presumes that naturally occurring reinforcers of stutter-free speech occur in the client's environment. The basic strategy is to attempt to foster in that environment many naturally occurring reinforcers, rather than the contrived or "unnatural" reinforcers that are associated with the clinic. The procedure usually involves verbal contingencies, and is particularly useful for cases of early stuttering where, as considered in later sections, verbal stimulation is likely to exert significant clinical control over stuttering. In such cases, relatives, family friends and preschool teachers are an indispensable component of treatment if they can provide verbal input as directed by a clinician.

Useful as it may be, it can be problematic to have persons other than immediate family providing input to a child's stuttering treatment. The reason is that the input can prove to be unhelpful, and may even traumatize the child. The clinician always needs to be on the lookout for negative, excessive, or uncontrolled sources of input. For example, an entire treatment program for a child can be disrupted if a preschool teacher directs attention to a child's speech in front of peers. It is a serious problem if a small child becomes negative about a treatment program. To avoid this, clinicians often delay input from non-family members until the treatment is well under way, and arrange for people other than the immediate family to avoid any kind of negative input and only praise the child for not stuttering. It is also worth noting that sibling rivalry can upset treatments for young children if siblings become "natural maintaining contingencies."

Natural maintaining contingencies have great value in the treatment of adults. This applies not only to reinforcement of stutter-free speech, but also for reinforcement of compliance with the treatment program, because treatments for adults can involve many laborious hours of speech practice. In order to complete the requirements of treatment, many adults who stutter require the support and encouragement from people around them. Some adult stuttering clients are well motivated and will succeed no matter what, but there are many who will not succeed if the only "maintaining contingencies" come from the clinician during clinic contacts. The clinician needs to enlist the support of family and friends.

## Train sufficient exemplars

This technique involves training the client in a few of the speech settings that are typical of the client's speaking life. This technique is nothing more than clinical commonsense; if the goal of treatment is to have the client stutter-free in everyday situations, then it does not make much sense to do all the training of stutter-free speech in a clinic which bears little resemblance to those situations. Perhaps a reason why treatment of early stuttering is so successful compared to treatment of advanced stuttering is that most of the treatment of young children is conducted by parents in everyday speaking situations.

In the case of adults, clinical settings encourage clinicians not to train sufficient exemplars, especially the intensive treatment format for stuttering. Although such treatments may use settings which are typical of the client's life in a program of sequential modification, stutter-free speech is usually taught wholly within the clinic at a time prior to that. It is possible that intensive prolonged speech treatments may achieve better generalization if stutter-free speech is trained in other situations in addition to the speech clinic. For example, clients might undergo prolonged speech training at home with a spouse, with a friend at that friend's house, or perhaps even with a trusted colleague at work.

## Train loosely

Discriminated learning is said to have occurred when stimuli associated with the treatment setting become stimuli for stutter-free speech.[1] Discriminated learning is an ever-present threat to the chances of achieving generalization (and therefore successful treatment). It would be expected that the chance of discriminated learning can be reduced by varying the settings, people and materials across treatment sessions. Home treatment sessions should not be conducted always in the same place, or with the same persons or materials. Instead, these features of the treatment can be systematically varied.

## Use indiscriminable reinforcers

This term refers to another way the clinician can prevent the occurrence of discriminated learning. By making the reinforcers unpredictable, it is more difficult for the client to discriminate learning to those reinforcers—they are made "indiscriminable." The technique is of most relevance with children. Of course, in early stages of treatment it is important for reinforcers to be predictable as a child learns to master stutter-free speech. However, continued predictability of this kind could be expected to hinder effective generalization; if a child expects reinforcers at a certain time or a certain place, that might encourage stutter-free speech only at that time or place. One procedure to incorporate unpredictable reinforcers in management is for a parent to assess a child covertly for a randomly chosen period during each day—say 10 minutes. The child is informed that such a surprise assessment will occur once each day, and at the conclusion of the assessment period the parent announces that an assessment has occurred and gives the result. If the child is within criterion performance (for example, "no stutters" or "less than two stutters"), a reinforcer is earned.

The technique of unexpected assessment is also useful for treatment of adults, especially if it is yoked to the treatment program. For example, a client may be able to pass a certain stage of the treatment program contingent on succeeding in a number of unpredictable assessments. Those assessments can be conducted by spouse or friends, or the clinician. One particularly effective method of unexpected assessment that a clinician can use is with the telephone. The client is informed that such assessments will occur, but has no idea when the clinician will telephone. During the telephone conversation, the clinician measures %SS and SPM on-line and the client is required to meet criterion performance in those measures. As is the case with the use of covert assessment (see page 46), there are some ethical issues associated with unexpected assessment and the client needs to agree to it in principle. Although some clients welcome the procedure as a challenge, it will be unsuitable for some clients because it causes them to be anxious.

## Program common stimuli

This is another technique that is particularly useful with children. It actually takes advantage of discriminated learning (see above). Stimuli from the child's environment are brought into the treatment setting in the hope that they will become discriminative stimuli for stutter-free speech. Obviously, one or both parents are powerful stimuli to have in the treatment setting, and it is difficult to imagine that treatment of childhood stuttering could be effective without such common stimuli. However, the technique can incorporate other kinds of stimuli. For example, a toy is nominated (or obtained specially) to be an accompaniment to treatment sessions. Cuddly toys, or "good talking badges" or special garments are particularly useful. Such stimuli can then accompany the child in everyday

---

[1] See the footnote on page 46. In this situation the rating machine is said to be a "discriminative stimulus."

speaking situations. For example, a child can have a "good talking badge" which is worn during treatment sessions and which is also worn during family outings to facilitate generalization of stutter-free speech.[1]

The technique of programming common stimuli may be applied also in treatment of adults if the client uses certain devices each day as part of treatment and if those devices become discriminated stimuli for stutter-free speech. Examples of such devices would be hand-held counters and small tape recorders, which are commonly used each day by clients during treatment. As mentioned previously (see footnote page 46), devices which a clinician uses in the clinic may cause discriminated learning with adults, so it makes sense to arrange things so that such learning has a chance to occur with objects which are not associated with the clinic. As is the case with children, common stimuli can include people from the adult client's daily environment. For example, it would be a potentially powerful aid to generalization if a client's spouse attended and participated in treatment sessions.

## Mediating generalization

This is where generalization is enhanced by having the client self-manage the continued production of the desired response. In other words, the response is brought under the internal control of the client rather than the external control of clinician, parents, reinforcers, and so on. Clinicians generally believe that self monitoring, self evaluation, and increased attention to the act of speech in general, may mediate generalization in clients of all ages. Reduced speech rate is another example of a mediator of generalization, although, as considered later, its clinical applications are quite limited. Arguably the mediators of generalization which are most used by clinicians are the speech patterns, or parts of the speech patterns, in prolonged speech treatments. The notion of mediating generalization raises the issue that stuttering is thought by some to be "incurable," (for example, see Cooper, 1987) and hence generalization will always need to be mediated. This viewpoint means that an adult client who learns to control stuttering will always need to self monitor and attend carefully to the act of speech, use prolonged speech, and so on. An alternative clinical viewpoint—or hope, or goal—is that the adult client will eventually be able to control the disorder with very little increased attention to speech.

## Train to generalize

As discussed previously, clinicians have much to gain from considering a number of client responses which may be useful in stuttering treatment. One of those responses is generalization, meaning that clinicians can simply train clients to generalize using techniques which they use to train clients to do other things. Again, it is only commonsense that what can be done to help a client achieve stutter-free speech can also be done to help a client *generalize* stutter-free speech. For example, RCS techniques (see page 48) can be used not only to reinforce stutter-free speech, but also to reinforce its generalization. The distinction between these two things can be quite subtle, but, especially with children, it is useful to recognize the difference between praising a child for speaking without stuttering and praising the child for doing so in an everyday situation.

---

[1] Parents can present a gift of such a toy at the first clinic visit. In addition to possibly contributing to generalization, this strategy can help the child to enjoy the visits to the clinic.

# The clinical functions of maintenance

If asked to list the most troublesome things about stuttering treatment, most clinicians would probably mention posttreatment relapse. Because of this it would be prudent, as suggested previously, to consider that the maintenance of stutter-free speech is a discrete treatment goal. The time that maintenance begins is not the point at which treatment ends. It is the start of the part of treatment where the client is trained in ways to keep the benefits of treatment in place for a long time. Helping clients to maintain stutter-free speech requires some specific clinician activities that do not occur at any other part of treatment. In the following sections some of those activities are considered.

## Promoting durable, stutter-free speech

This is one of the most obvious goals of maintenance in stuttering treatment. Unfortunately, it is not obvious what clinical procedures should be used to achieve it. Although posttreatment relapse is a particularly daunting treatment problem with this disorder, there has been very little research into how clinicians might overcome that problem. An experiment by Ingham (1980) provided one useful clue by showing how maintenance can be conceptualized as a treatment goal, and how programmed instruction can be used to train that goal. Ingham studied nine clients who had just completed a sequential modification procedure for generalization (see above). The subjects were divided into two groups. For one group, maintenance was administered in a performance-contingent schedule of clinic visits (see page 62). The other group received a non-performance-contingent schedule where clients attended the clinic at regular intervals regardless of their performance in the previous session. It was found that the performance contingent schedule was associated with better group maintenance than the non-performance-contingent schedule. In other words, the performance contingent schedule of speech assessments reinforced the maintenance of stutter-free speech. The details of this maintenance procedure will be considered shortly.

## Facilitating client and/or parent management responsibility

If the goal of stuttering treatment is to acquire stutter-free speech and keep it for a long period of time, then one thing is obvious. To achieve such a goal, at some time clients or clients and their parents need to assume the responsibility for the management of their disorder. The resources of speech pathologists are too limited to have all their clients dependent on them for maintenance of their stutter-free speech.[1] Accordingly, it is recommended that all client or parent contacts during the maintenance phase of treatments are structured to facilitate the transfer of management responsibility to clients or clients and their parents.

One simple way to achieve this goal is to base maintenance procedures entirely or substantially on speech performance measures which are collected by clients/parents from outside the clinic. Another way to achieve this goal is to equip clients with a set of procedures to follow in the event of impending relapse. One useful procedure is to instruct clients in a set of steps to follow which are designed to restore stutter-free speech. The

---

[1] As with many disorders, peer support groups exist for people who stutter. Such groups are obviously an important resource for speech pathologists, and their role in stuttering treatment is considered in Part Six.

client/parent contacts the clinician in the event that relapse remains a problem after these steps have been followed.[1]

## Systematic removal of beyond-clinic controls over stuttering

At the time when the maintenance part of treatment is about to begin, the client will be engaged in many activities which contribute to the control of stuttered speech. One of the goals of maintenance is to remove those controls so that stutter-free speech is as effortless as is possible for the client. The clinician can use the maintenance part of treatment to determine exactly what level of control each client will require.

The template of a maintenance program presented in Table 2 shows one way that systematic removal of speech controls can be accomplished. The technique is for the client to be assessed frequently at the start of maintenance, but for assessments to gradually become less frequent on the condition that treatment gains remain in place. Another way that systematic removal of speech controls can occur is when clients or parents conduct activities on a daily basis as part of the treatment. For example, an adult client may perform speech drills each day which are designed to ensure that the client retains the skill of using a speech pattern to eliminate stuttered speech. That speech practice could be withdrawn systematically throughout the maintenance program as follows. After a month of maintenance, speech drills can be conducted for six days of each week. If speech performance does not deteriorate, then for the next month speech drills can be conducted for five days of each week. If speech performance still does not deteriorate, then speech practice can occur on four days of each week, and so on until the point is found at which treatment gains remain in place with the minimum practice.

### Detection of relapse

In any disorder where relapse may occur, effective management depends on the detection of relapse as soon as it occurs. This is an important goal of maintenance activities. If a client becomes stutter-free but then begins to relapse, it is far better if intervention occurs immediately than if it occurs some months, or even some years later. Adult clients often present to a clinician after they have relapsed subsequent to an intensive treatment program. This means that the client is experiencing the effect of the disorder again, and the clinician has to start almost from scratch with a new treatment. In the case of young children, it is particularly important to detect any signs of relapse because the passage of time could result in the disorder becoming less tractable.

### Support

Kirschenbaum and Tomarken (1977) draw attention to the fact that people may have difficulty maintaining positive behavior change, no matter how beneficial it is for them. No matter how much better someone feels after losing weight, stopping smoking, or exercising, there is always a tendency to relapse to the previous behaviors. Stuttering treatment is no exception. Counselling is an important contribution to helping people maintain the stutter-free spech they have acquired through their treatment.

---

[1] A similar strategy is used in the management of many medical conditions. For example, at the start of an attack, the client follows a prescribed set of procedures, and seeks medical attention if those procedures do not control the attack.

# Speech performance criteria for maintenance

Relapse may occur so often simply because the maintenance part of treatment is the longest. In other words, things may go wrong simply because there is so much time for them to go wrong. To the clinician, this means that there is all the more reason to get things right, and one of the best ways to get maintenance right is not to conceptualize it as a haphazard "follow-up" or "review" procedure. As argued previously, it is worthwhile to think of maintenance as a treatment goal that is trained systematically. The following sections outline how speech measures and programmed instruction can be used to do that.

Speech measures in maintenance are used to specify what is to be accepted as satisfactory speech, and are chosen with the needs of the individual client in mind. In many cases, some of the following measures will not be suitable, or will be modified in some fashion.

## Within-clinic %SS

At each clinic visit during maintenance the client speaks a specified number of syllables to the clinician and %SS is measured on-line during a 5- or 10-minute conversation. The client does not pass the maintenance visit if a criterion number of stutters is exceeded for the conversation. The number of syllables spoken during this procedure depends on the type and age of client.[1] The benefit of the procedure is that the client speaks face-to-face with the clinician, and can notice things that cannot be noticed on tape recordings of the client speaking outside the clinic. For example, during the within-clinic conversation the clinician may notice things that suggest the client is struggling a great deal to prevent stuttered speech. If the criterion for within-clinic %SS in maintenance is not met, then the client returns to the first step of the maintenance program (see below).

## Beyond-clinic %SS or SMST

This measure is identical in all respects to within-clinic %SS, except that it is based on tape recorded conversations of the client in a variety of daily situations. As part of maintenance activities, the client or parent collects the tape recordings and presents them to the clinician at designated times. These measures can be the backbone of structured maintenance. In many cases—hopefully most cases—the client or the parent can be trained to assess these tape recordings for %SS so that the clinician does not have to spend time on these measurements. Having clients or parents measure speech performance has the additional advantage, as discussed previously, of facilitating the transfer of management responsibility to them. On many occasions the clinician will instruct the client/parent in collecting of SMST measures because they are simpler to master than %SS measures. It is recommended during maintenance that a number of beyond-clinic %SS or SMST measures are collected in the week prior to the maintenance assessment. As with within-clinic %SS, the client returns to the first step of the maintenance program if the maintenance criterion for beyond-clinic %SS is not met (see below).

## Unexpected telephone call

If speaking on the telephone without stuttering is a treatment goal, then this is a particularly effective form of maintenance assessment. It may be used with all adult clients,

---

[1] The actual amount of speech that is sampled depends on how much is needed to satisfy the clinician that a valid measure of the client's speech is being gathered. That may take several hundred or several thousand syllables.

and for any children who will converse readily on the telephone. Sometime during the week prior to the maintenance visit, the clinician telephones unexpectedly and speaks to the client. The clinician measures %SS on-line, and the client does not pass the forthcoming maintenance visit if a criterion measure is exceeded. The clinician may wish parents to conduct this procedure with their child, or the spouse of a client to conduct the procedure. For example, a parent could telephone the child from work and collect SMST measures on-line.

There are several reservations about the surprise telephone call technique. The first is that the privacy of the client needs to be respected. The technique is not feasible unless the client agrees to it and arrangements are made about when calls will and will not be made. The second reservation is that stuttering may be more difficult to detect over the telephone than they are in real time or from tape recordings.

### Beyond-clinic severity ratings

In a previous section it was argued that a 10-point stuttering severity scale, based on five minutes of conversational speech, was an accessible and convenient measurement procedure for very young clients. During maintenance, that measure provides a convenient way to prescribe criterion performance for a child. It is recommended that during the week prior to each maintenance visit, the parent records a severity rating (or several severity ratings) each day according to procedures described on page 42. The child does not pass the maintenance assessment if a criterion mean severity rating score is exceeded. For example, a child may be required to achieve a severity score of 2.2 or less. If that criterion is not met, the child returns to the first step in the maintenance program (see below). The value of maintenance activities will depend on the representativeness of the chosen speaking situations, and also on the reliability of the parent in using the severity scale.

# A template for programmed instruction in maintenance

As discussed earlier, the basic clinical approach to maintenance is to consider it a required client response, in the same way that stutter-free speech is regarded as a required client response. One procedure is to reward clients or clients and parents for successful maintenance. The reward for lasting for a certain period of time without relapse can be for the next assessment to occur after a longer period of time. In other words, each successful maintenance assessment "earns" a longer period of time until the next visit. A hypothetical maintenance program, consisting of eight steps, is presented in Table 2. This program is adapted from Ingham (1980; 1987a). Any unsuccessful maintenance visit results in a return to the first maintenance step (M1).[1] Maintenance programs are constructed according to the needs of individual clients and their families; the number of maintenance steps, the time period between each step, and the performance criteria all vary from client to client.

Success in the maintenance program means fewer assessments, because beyond-clinic measures are made only in the week preceding visits. The total duration of the program shown in Table 2 will be 66 weeks if no failure occurs at any step. However, some failure

---

[1] A variation on this procedure which is appropriate in some situations is to permit one failure at any step of the maintenance program. Should such a failure occur, the client or parent and child return the following week and attempt again to meet the requirements of that maintenance step. If a second failure occurs, then the the client or parent and child return to the first step in the maintenance program.

should be anticipated at some point point during maintenance. Changing performance criteria to prevent a client failing a step could have disastrous consequences for the success of the program. The temptation to do so can be great, especially when a client fails by a small margin, such as when a child achieves a mean severity score of 2.1 when the criterion is 2.0. Of course, there will be occasions when criteria should be altered during a maintenance program to prevent a client from failing a step, but to do so without a good reason defeats the purpose of programmed maintenance instruction. If a client does not succeed in meeting maintenance criteria, then a return to more frequent clinic contact is necessary for maintenance to continue successfully.

TABLE TWO: A hypothetical maintenance program, adapted from Ingham (1987)

| Step | Weeks to next step | Pass: Go To | Fail: Go To |
|------|-----|-----|-----|
| M1 | 1 | M2 | M1 |
| M2 | 1 | M3 | M1 |
| M3 | 2 | M4 | M1 |
| M4 | 2 | M5 | M1 |
| M5 | 4 | M6 | M1 |
| M6 | 8 | M7 | M1 |
| M7 | 16 | M8 | M1 |
| M8 | 32 | - | M1 |

As with all treatments in speech pathology, it is not wise to allow a high failure rate. If a client—especially a child—repeatedly fails to meet the requirements of a maintenance program and returns to the first step, that client may require further training in the skill of producing stutter-free speech. To do this, the clinician may postpone the maintenance program until the client has obtained those necessary skills.

## Using the telephone in maintenance

Telephone headsets and hands-free telephones are useful equipment during maintenance. There is no doubt that all clients require some clinician contact during maintenance, especially when there is substantial counselling to be done. But in many cases it is not necessary for the client or the client and parents to attend the clinic for all maintenance visits. On some occasions, all that is needed is the client's voice over the telephone and the client's beyond-clinic speech measures. It might even be counterproductive for the child and parent to attend all maintenance visits, because it may discourage client or parent responsibility for maintenance. Also, in some respects, a telephone conversation with the clinician is a more valid speech measure than a within-clinic conversation. This procedure will not be suitable for children who are unwilling to converse with the clinician on the telephone, or clients whose stuttering requires visual inspection to be detected.

With the program outlined in Table 2, clinic visits might be scheduled at M4 and M8 only. Of course, the client/parent can visit the clinic on any maintenance assessment date if the need arises. The remainder of the maintenance assessments could then be conducted by telephone. On the date of the maintenance assessment, the clinician could telephone and collect %SS on-line in place of a within-clinic measure. If they are used in maintenance, severity ratings are conveyed to the clinician by the parent during this conversation. If beyond-clinic %SS or SMST data are collected by the client or parent, those data are also conveyed to the clinician. If the clinician checks the client/parent's %SS or SMST data from tape recordings, the clinician must receive recordings by mail prior to the date of the maintenance assessment. On the basis of these data, the client either passes or fails that maintenance step. During this telephone contact, it is important to discuss progress with the client/parent and initiate any counselling in the same fashion as would occur at a clinic visit.

# Part Three:

# Management of
# Early Stuttering

# The Distinctiveness of Early Stuttering

In this text the term "early stuttering" refers to children who have begun to stutter in the preschool years, most commonly in the second or third year of life, and who have been stuttering for a short period of from one to three years. Early stuttering has some features which distinguish it from advanced stuttering. These distinguishing features have profound implications for clinical management, so they are considered in the sections below.

## Responsiveness to intervention

Many clinicians have observed that early stuttering is far more responsive to intervention than advanced stuttering (Adams, 1984; Bloodstein, 1987; Costello, 1983; Curlee, 1984; 1993; Ingham, 1984; Prins, 1983; Riley & Riley, 1983; Starkweather, 1990; St. Louis & Westbrook, 1987). Curlee (1993) states that

> it is widely believed that identification and appropriate clinical intervention with young incipient stutterers comprise the most effective management strategy for preventing stuttering from becoming a chronic, long-term disability. (p. 1)

Some data are available which indicate that early stuttering can be controlled in quite short periods of time (Martin, Kuhl, & Haroldson, 1972; Onslow, Costa, & Rue, 1990; Reed & Godden, 1970). Martin, Kuhl, and Haroldson (1972) controlled the stuttering of two preschool-age children in a few short laboratory sessions, and Onslow, Costa, and Rue (1990) reported that an effective treatment for four preschool-age stuttering children required from 5 to 8 hours of clinician time. A report by Onslow, Andrews, and Lincoln (in press) presented treatment time data for a caseload of 12 children younger than 5 years. The children reached target performance criteria in a mean of 11.5 clinic sessions, with a range of 5-22 sessions.

In contrast to early stuttering, advanced stuttering is generally less tractable (Cooper, 1987; Ingham & Onslow, 1987; Martin, 1981; Van Riper, 1973), and treatment programs require more clinician time per client (Ingham, 1984; Starkweather, 1990). This is partly because many cases of advanced stuttering relapse to stuttered speech some time after treatment, and those relapsed clients may require further treatment.[1] Clinicians frequently encounter adult clients seeking treatment who have been treated at some time previously. In contrast to this, it is generally believed that maintenance of treatment gains with early stuttering involves less effort.

---

[1] There have been several attempts to assess how many cases of advanced stuttering relapse after treatment. However, it would be misleading to cite a general figure for this because of the many different ways that relapse might be defined. Arguably, though, posttreatment relapse is the most serious problem with treatment of advanced stuttering.

# Variability and periods of remission

It is generally believed that early stuttering occurs in episodes. It can cease completely for periods and then start again. Johnson and Associates (1959) reported that 34.7 percent of mothers of stuttering preschool children felt that stuttering had "completely disappeared" at some time. According to survey data presented by Onslow, Harrison and Jones (1993), 41.4 percent of parents of stuttering children responded similarly. Additionally, extreme variations in severity over short periods are well known to clinicians who treat children who have recently begun to stutter. Such variations can occur even in a single day. Johnson and Associates reported that 73.2 percent of parents of preschool stuttering children said that there was a time when the child's speech "improved greatly." [1]

The episodic nature of early stuttering has been described by many clinicians (Bloodstein, 1987, Ingham, 1993; Curlee, 1993; Luper & Mulder, 1964; Onslow, Harrison, & Jones, 1992; Peters & Guitar, 1991; Starkweather, Gottwald, & Halfond, 1990; Van Riper, 1971; Wingate, 1976). Wingate (1976) and Curlee (1993) note that preschool-age stuttering children may present to a clinic but show no signs of stuttered speech. A common scenario is for a concerned parent to contact a speech clinic because a child has begun to stutter, and for the child to be placed on a waiting list for assessment. However, when the clinic contacts the parent to arrange an appointment, the parent reports that stuttering has stopped. Yet that parent recontacts the clinic some time later and reports that stuttering has begun again. Van Riper (1971) reports of his extensive clinical experiences that

> in most instances, the younger the stutterer, the more he tended to oscillate from one level of severity to another. Periods characterized by many syllabic repetitions on many words alternated with other periods as long as a week or month when only two or three such repetitions occurred per day...Developmentally the severity of stuttering seems to see-saw back and forth. Sometimes on the backswing, the stutterer may become completely fluent for days. (p. 103)

In addition to being episodic, early stuttering seems to be particularly variable, as shown in data reported by Onslow, Andrews, and Costa (1990). Onslow et al. collected daily speech samples from four preschool-age children for around three weeks, and for each subject, the number of stutters per sample counted by a clinician ranged as follows: 0-17, 1-30, 2-16, 3-26.

# Recovery without formal intervention

As mentioned several times in previous sections, some cases of early stuttering recover without formal treatment from a speech pathologist. Again, this is a distinguishing feature of the early stages of the disorder. If it persists into adulthood, then it is not likely to disappear "spontaneously." Instead, it is likely that help from a speech pathologist will be necessary to eliminate stuttered speech.

# Interpreting the distinctiveness of early stuttering

The above three observations about the differences between early and advanced stuttering are of enormous interest. They suggest that early stuttering is a far more tractable condition than advanced stuttering; it responds better to treatment, it can disappear

---

[1] They also reported responses to the same question asked of a group of parents of nonstuttering children who had normal disfluencies. Interestingly, only 23.7 percent of those parents reported that the normal disfluencies were "improved greatly" at some time.

completely for periods, and it may remit without formal treatment. This information suggests a lot about the kind of treatment which might be suitable for early stuttering. This matter is addressed in the following paragraphs.

One way of viewing the clinical process with stuttering clients is as a process of skill acquisition. Hopefully, the client will achieve the skill necessary for stutter-free speech. Bellack and Hersen (1977) offer some useful insights into problem behaviors of children in terms of skill deficit. First, problem behaviors may exist because of a skill decicit. In other words, someone may not have the skills required to produce the desired behavior, and so an undesired behavior is produced instead. In communication disorders, an example would be errors of articulation; a child produces the undesired behavior (articulation error) simply because the child is unable to produce the desirable behavior (correct articulation).

The second of Bellack and Hersen's explanations for the existence of childhood problem behaviors is that the child may have the skill to produce the desired behavior, but insufficient prompts for that behavior come from the child's environment. An example of a desirable behavior of early childhood is saying "thank you" when given something by an adult (see page 49). Obviously, most children are able to say "thank you" when they are given something. Equally obvious is that many of them fail to do this. So, when children fail to say "thank you," it may be only because they are not prompted to say it. Bellack and Hersen point out that a child in this situation may not even be aware that "thank you" is a desirable response.

The third of Bellack and Hersen's explanations for problem childhood behavior is that the child has the skill to produce the desired response, which is prompted and appears, but is not maintained because its occurrence is not reinforced. Using the "thank you" example, a parent may prompt a child to say this, which elicits the response on several occasions. However the response may quickly disappear if the parent fails to reinforce this desirable behavior when it occurs on other occasions.

Bellack and Hersen's perspective indicates that childhood behavior problems do not necessarily reflect an underlying skill deficit. Such problems may occur even though the child is capable of producing the desired behavior. The implication of this for managing early stuttering is that young children who stutter may be quite capable of producing stutter-free speech. The distinctiveness of early stuttering reviewed in previous paragraphs strongly suggests that this is so; (1) early stuttering is more tractable than advanced stuttering, (2) it can remit for substantial periods of time and (3) children can recover from it without formal treatment. These features are consistent with stutter-free speech being within the behavioral repertoire of young children. A clinician may be justified in assuming that older-age clients really do have a skill deficit and are incapable of producing stutter-free speech. But it would be extremely incautious to assume that this is the case for early stuttering.

It might be concluded, then, that early stuttering is quite an innocuous condition compared to advanced stuttering, and it probably has in common with many behavior problems of childhood that it does not involve a skill deficit. Therefore, the first treatment of choice for early stuttering recommended here is an operant approach which incorporates techniques that parents generally use to manage the behavior of their young children. The justification for this first choice of treatment for early stuttering is discussed in detail in Part Seven, along with its various shortcomings. The arguments in favor of an operant approach to early stuttering can be summarized by stating that it is the simplest and the conceptually soundest approach that is available, and that operant methodology has been shown empirically to control stuttering.

# Eliminating
# Stuttered Speech

## Overview

The techniques for eliminating early stuttering outlined in this section were reported by Onslow, Costa, and Rue (1990). They incorporate RCS (operant methodology; see Part Two) which is provided by parents. The clinician models the procedures in the clinic and trains parents in using those procedures. Parents then administer the procedures in their children's everyday speaking environments. Procedures are administered both in *sessions* and *on-line* , and may be accompanied by clinical activities and materials that are suitable for young children. At all times, the clinician is mindful of the important ethical issues that surround the use of operant interventions with young children.[1]

## Parenting and operant methodology with young children

Bellack and Hersen (1977) state that operant techniques are particularly effective with problem behaviors of childhood, and that one reason for this is that parents control a number of potent reinforcers for children. Probably the most potent of these are approval and affection, which children associate with comfort and security. To that might be added that contingency management is essentially an extension of common practices which parents use to control various problem behaviors in children. Therefore the training of parents in contingency management procedures for stuttering is often straightforward. Most parents will be able to relate to the idea that a child's problem behavior can be changed with consistent feedback to the child.

A supportive and constructive environment which contains consistent feedback is essential for a child to learn stutter-free speech. However some parents may not readily provide that environment, in which case a clinician needs to spend time training parents to do so. A related problem can occur in families where both parents work and there are other young children. The effort of caring for a young family, combined with occupational stresses, can leave little time or energy for a treatment program as extensive as that required to manage early stuttering.

Some parents are not accustomed to showing pleasure at their child's efforts and improvements. If that is the case, then it requires attention from the clinician in order for an RCS treatment for stuttering to be effective. It is also the case that some parents may experience negative feelings about their child's stuttering. Added to other life stresses associated with a young family, the stuttered speech of a child can be frustrating or irritating for parents. In which case, a clinician needs to address how they might handle such negative

---

[1] The outline of an RCS treatment for early stuttering in the following sections is intended neither as a detailed manual of clinical procedures nor as an aid to clinical instruction.

feelings about the child's speech in an appropriate fashion that will not interfere with the treatment. Sometimes, inadvertent communication of negative messages to the child about speech will undermine the effectiveness of a treatment. It is also the case that many parents have been misinformed—based on outdated approaches to the disorder (see Part Two)—that any direct attention to their child's stuttering will be harmful. This can cause anxiety and make parents reluctant to participate in a treatment where attention is drawn directly to the child's stuttered speech. Correcting such misinformation is often an important task for the clinician.

It is difficult to conduct a behaviorally-based treatment program for stuttering if parents fail to exert control over the general behavior of a child. This may occur because the behavior of some children is difficult to control. It may also occur that a child has been "perfect" in the first years of life, and consequently the parents have never needed to exert substantive control over behavior. Then, with the onset of stuttering, they are confronted with a situation in which they require considerable compliance from a child in achieving behavior change. The result can be that such parents have no effective strategies for obtaining the cooperation necessary for the treatment.

Cases occur where the clinician finds that a suitable environment for learning stutter-free speech cannot be established without professional team management. In such cases the clinician may wish to explore with parents the possible need for external involvement, and perhaps make an appropriate referral. Examples might involve tensions within the household, a parent with serious emotional difficulties, or a child who has severe behavioral disturbances.

## Ethics and operant methodology with young children

Bellack and Hersen (1977) discuss the important issue of ethics and the use of operant methodology with young children. An initial point of concern of those authors is that, in the case of very young clients, it is a person other than the client who determines that intervention is desirable and determines whether an intervention has been satisfactory. The client is "not free to determine what, if anything, they want from treatment or when it should end" (p. 208). Generally, it is clear that elimination of stuttered speech is in the interests of the child. However, the clinician must be absolutely sure that all aspects of the treatment are beneficial to the child rather than serving the interests of some other person. Bellack and Hersen indicate that this is a common misuse of operant methodology with children. For example, it would be inappropriate to impose unusually stringent criteria for treatment success because a child's parents were particularly demanding people.

Another issue touched on by Bellack and Hersen is more directly relevant to stuttering treatment; the use of tangible reinforcers. Those authors state that the nature of such reinforcers—extrinsic rather than intrinsic to the client—has prompted considerable controversy. They cite the following objections that have been raised:

> it is bribery; it teaches greed; it reduces the effectiveness of alternative (natural) means of control;....good behavior should be intrinsically rewarding...token reinforcement systems reduce intrinsic interest in tasks so reinforced. (p. 209)

Bellack and Hersen argue that such notions apply only when tangible reinforcement is used "inappropriately, excessively, or in isolation," (p. 209) but not when tangible reinforcers are used appropriately. If such an argument is valid, it suggests that it is the responsibility of clinicians to properly understand and utilize the principles of tangible reinforcement.

The final ethical consideration raised by Bellack and Hersen (1977) relates to punishment. In the case of stuttering, as with many problems of childhood, punishment is particularly effective. However,

> of all behavioral techniques, punishment has the greatest likelihood of misuse. Many people find it easier to apply punishment than to expend the effort to identify and apply positive reinforcement procedures for behavior incompatible with the undesired response. Punishment is also attractive because its impact is often more quickly visible than the effects of positive reinforcement. Finally, punishment can be a form of aggression and retribution, which are frequently the natural responses to the anger engendered by undesirable child behavior. (p. 209)

In short, there is good cause to be concerned that incorrect parental use of punishment could cause significant harm to a young child. The ethics of the speech pathology profession require clinicians to consider the well being of the client paramount. Therefore, there is a need to be particularly vigilant in the monitoring of parents' use of verbal punishment procedures. In particular, under no circumstances should a clinician recommend the use of verbal punishment procedures for early stuttering until there is excellent reason to believe that the parents concerned are capable of administering this procedure as intended by the clinician. Further, when a clinician instigates a program that involves negative verbal stimulation, it is necessary to ensure that the clinician accurately monitors the use of such stimulation by parents. At the least, the clinician should directly observe the parents' negative verbal stimulation in the clinic, and monitor parents' negative verbal stimulation beyond the clinic by means of tape recordings of that stimulation being administered beyond the clinic. These simple procedures can detect errors that parents often make in delivering negative stimulation to their children. Failure to use such procedures is inconsistent with the ethics of the speech pathology profession.

# Reinforcement

Bellack and Hersen (1977) state the crucial principle that all behavioral interventions for young children focus on reinforcement. The commonsense in this principle is evident: Efforts to change the behavior of a very young child are not likely to succeed unless feedback focuses mostly on what is done correctly, rather than on what is done incorrectly. In the case of management of early stuttering, this suggests a focus primarily on stutter-free speech. Obviously, most 2- and 3-year-old children will respond adversely to feedback which emphasizes the occurrence of stuttering. One of the most serious problems in the management of early stuttering is for the child to react adversely to treatment because it is a negative experience overall. Being negative can ruin any human interaction, and it is a guarantee of failure in attempts to modify the stuttering of a young child.

Bellack and Hersen cite the useful "Grandma's Rule" as a procedure for applying reinforcement in any treatment format. First, a prompt specifies or reiterates the correct behavior and the contingency, then the reinforcer is given when the desirable behavior appears. In other words, tell the child what you want to happen and what the reward will be if it happens, and then give the reward when it does happen.

## The reinforcer

It is critical to select reinforcers which are suitable for the individual child. This selection is normally based on consultation with the child and parent/s, and on clinical trial-and-error. Four classes of reinforcer cited by Bellack and Hersen are:

1. Primary reinforcers (e.g. food, drink).
2. Social reinforcers (e.g. attention and approval).
3. Desired activities and tangible materials (e.g. money, toys, special outings).
4. Tokens; stimuli that represents any of the above three reinforcers (e.g. stamps, stickers, chain links, stars on the fridge). These are of value because of their convenience and their appeal to young children.

Bellack and Hersen cite the following crucial principles to follow when using reinforcement:

1. The reinforcer is not available to the child in any other context but treatment.
2. When the reinforcer is administered at a high rate, small portions are necessary to avoid satiation.
3. At the start of intervention, the reinforcer occurs immediately after every response (period of stutter-free speech). However, systematic variation of this schedule is crucial to the success of the intervention.
4. If a partially adequate response occurs initially, successive approximations are reinforced.
5. To ensure the child's continued interest in them, many different reinforcers are used over a period of time.

# Punishment

The lay concept of punishment tends to emphasize the stimulus rather than its effects on the behavior in question. For example, a smack is often considered by parents to be a punishment, when, strictly speaking, a smack could only be considered a punishment if it reduced the occurrence of a problem behavior. Of itself, a smack is merely a negative thing. Because of this potential confusion about punishment, it might be advisable when dealing with parents of young children to avoid the use of the word "punishment." Bellack and Hersen (1977) also state that it is unwise to use punishment as a sole treatment technique, and that it should not be used unless it is necessary. When trialing a procedure involving punishment, abandon it immediately if the child shows any aversion to it. Many children respond favorably to punishment, but many do not.

## Application of negative stimulation

Negative stimulation with properties likely to be unpleasant to children—especially direct, tangible varieties—has no place in stuttering treatment.[1] Verbal punishment is the most commonly used negative stimulation that is applied to young children. This involves drawing attention to stuttering when it occurs, and, on some occasions, requesting the child to repeat the utterance without stuttering. A technique that may be used in association with this process is *overcorrection,,* where the child is asked to repeat the correct behavior a

---

[1] In the case of some serious behavioral problems of childhood, the use of unpleasant stimuli might be justified, but certainly never for the treatment of stuttering.

number of times. This procedure makes sense because it can transform the child's experience of receiving negative stimulation into a positive experience because the correct response occurs more than the original error response. For this reason, overcorrection can be a useful strategy when a child makes several attempts to correct a stuttered utterance before achieving success.

## Withdrawal of reinforcing stimulation

This is a much favored form of punishment because it circumvents the problems associated with applying negative stimulation to children. Instead, positive stimulation is withdrawn contingent on stuttering. Below are presented two variations of punishment by contingent withdrawal of stimulation:

1. Response cost, where a positive reinforcer is surrendered contingent on stuttering. This procedure is used mostly in conjunction with token systems.
2. Time-out (TO), where the child is removed from a source of positive reinforcement. With rare exceptions, this procedure is not suitable for young children.

# Treatment Formats

## Treatment in sessions

The child and parent/s spend time together at regular intervals in a structured setting, when procedures to produce stutter-free speech are applied. Generally between 5 and 30 minutes is a suitable duration, although on many occasions the parent stops the session when a child fatigues or loses interest. The predominant technique used is verbal stimulation. This consists of reinforcement, sometimes combined with punishment. Tangible reinforcers are used, as appropriate to the child.[1] Story books can be used as stimuli, or the sessions can be based on conversation. It is not possible to recommend a duration or frequency of these sessions. Different durations and frequencies of sessions will be suitable for different families.

The clinician designs the procedures to be used in home sessions, trains the parent/s in their application, and monitors the administration of the sessions. As mentioned above, an important rule is never to recommend that sessions are conducted at home until (1) parent/s have been observed conducting them effectively in the clinic and (2) tape recorded evidence is heard showing that sessions are conducted properly in the home. Otherwise, a great deal of treatment effort from the parents may be wasted, or the treatment may be unpleasant for the child.

The point of treatment in a session format is to provide a situation where it is easy for the child to produce stutter-free speech. Treatment might be conducted for the purpose of training stutter-free speech, or they may be conducted merely to provide tasks for the child in which success is sure to occur. Speech drills of this kind may not be necessary at all in some cases, and always at some point during the treatment this treatment format becomes unnecessary. There is no point in persisting with treatment sessions when they no longer contribute to the goal of stutter-free speech or when they no longer contribute to the child's confidence or motivation.

## Treatment on-line

Many cases of early stuttering can be managed solely with on-line verbal stimulation contingent on stuttered and stutter-free speech. In other cases, for all or part of the period of management, treatment sessions may be a necessary adjunct. Situations chosen for giving on-line feedback are chosen carefully. It may not be desirable, for example, to comment on a child's speech performance in the presence of peers.

Clinicians seem to agree that the value of on-line contingent verbal stimulation rests on it being given *consistently* throughout each day. The child receives feedback about speech at all times. However it is critical not to confuse "consistent" feedback with "frequent" feedback. Consistent feedback can occur at a rate of only once each hour. Providing excessive amounts

---

[1] The success of these sessions depends a lot on how effectively the parents can arrange activities that provide a continual source of interest to the child. Young children have little task orientation, but generally participate in tasks that are enjoyable.

of on-line feedback is likely to make the child bewildered and apprehensive about the intervention.

The child is given verbal stimulation (feedback), consisting of mostly reinforcement, during everyday speaking situations. Feedback consists of comments made about either specific stutters and specific periods free of stuttering, or comments made generally about speech performance. Feedback for specific instances of stuttering and stutter-free speech can occur for predetermined time intervals, such as for 10 minutes of every hour, twice a day for 10 minutes, for 2 hours of every day, and so on. Alternatively, on-line feedback can be given during a variety of predetermined situations, such as while shopping, in the car on the way to kindergarten, at Grandma's house, bath times, meal times, and so on. Another approach is for parents to provide feedback whenever they think it is appropriate during each day. The best frequency of feedback for stuttering, and the best times for it to occur, is different for each child. Appropriate methods for every child are established by the clinician through experimentation and consultation with parents.

The use of on-line verbal punishment is applied with *extreme caution.* It is the responsibility of the clinician to ensure that no client is exposed to excessive levels of negative verbal stimulation. Again, it is not ethical for clinicians to permit on-line feedback to occur without good reason to believe that parents can perform the task correctly.

Only in exceptional circumstances would it be advisable for a person not trained by the clinician to give on-line feedback to a child. The use of people in the child's customary speaking environment is a sound way to attempt to achieve generalization, as has been discussed previously, but it can create problems (see Part Two). Desirable as the contribution of additional persons are to treatment of young children, ethical considerations compel the clinician to ensure that such contributions are carefully defined, trained and monitored.

Onslow, Costa, and Rue (1990) present the following example of a parent's feedback to a child for stuttered speech and stutter-free speech. In this example, the parent identifies a stutter and requests the child to repeat the utterance without the stutter. The parent then overcorrects the error. This interaction could occur as a part of feedback on-line or in a session:

(Child)    "Mummy, that's a b-b-b-big doggy."
           (Referring to a picture book)

(Mother)   "Whoops, that was a bumpy word there. Try it again."

(Child)    "A big doggy."

(Mother)   "Very good, no bumpy words! Say it again!"

(Child)    "A big doggy"

(Mother)   "Good boy. You can do it without bumpy words, can't you? Say 'a big doggy' again."

(Child)    "Big doggy."

(Mother)   "Good boy." (Onslow, Costa, & Rue, 1990, p. 408)

# Programmed treatment

In some cases, the clinician may choose to administer the operant treatment described above with programmed instruction. This might be an option when success does not occur with a nonprogrammed approach. Such an approach might be chosen when preschool-age children present to clinicians with a history of failed treatment. Sometimes the clinician will interpret that history as a suggestion that a nonprogrammed approach is unlikely to be effective. Clinicians might also consider this approach in cases where a child's stuttering is severe. For example, a clinician may feel that a child with a stuttering rate of 20 %SS, with long blocks and prolongations, may benefit from a more systematic approach to achieving stutter-free speech.

The type of programmed instruction suitable for preschool childen is different to that normally used with older clients. As a group, young children have limited task orientation, less concentration span and less resistance to failure at treatment tasks than do older clients. Therefore, the programmed instruction attempted with young children needs to be a modified version of that used with older clients. The nature of those modifications is summarized below:

1. Instruction sessions are shorter than for adults. For a young child, 10 to 20 minutes might be the maximum period. If necessary, one way to compensate for this is to conduct more than one programmed instruction session each day.

2. Contingencies for errors are used with more flexibility. With a young child it is not always possible to stay with the same reinforcement schedule during a programmed instruction session. The parent who conducts the session needs to constantly watch the child for change of mood, and respond if necessary by changing the schedule of reinforcement, and perhaps the reinforcer itself.

3. The hierarchial sequence of treatment targets is constructed with ad hoc flexibility. For example, if the ELU program (see page 49) was adapted for a preschool-age child, it could not be used in the same form as with adults. Flexible adaptation of programmed instruction procedures for young children is a creative skill. For example, in the early stages of an ELU program, the child could be required to name increasing numbers of picture cards, or could be required to complete sentence repetition tasks for sentences of increasing duration. At later stages of the program, the parent can target stutter-free picture-book descriptions or conversations of increasing duration. An important point to note here is that, although treatment sessions are programmed, the child would normally receive nonprogrammed verbal RCS in customary speaking situations.

4. Negative contingencies are de-emphasized, because small children generally tolerate fewer of them than older clients. This is not an inflexible rule, because some children will respond well to negative stimulation and improve their performance accordingly. But generally it can cause problems if too many negative contingencies are used with small children.

# Treatment Targets

The following sections consider the material about treatment targets presented in Part Two with reference to the use of those targets with preschool-age children. Parents often ask whether they should say the words "stutter" and "stuttering" to their child during the treatment program. The answer depends on the individual child and parent. For some parent-child combinations it is best to use these words, and in other cases other words are appropriate.[1] The terms "bumpy words" or "stuck words" are often favored by parents to describe stuttering. Perhaps the most important consideration in choosing words to use in treatment of young children is that those words communicate clearly to the child about the undesirable behaviour. For example, if a child perceived that speech becomes "stuck" when stuttering, the term "stuck word" might be useful during treatment.

## Stutter-free speech

Stutter-free speech is a particularly useful treatment focus with young children who stutter because it gives the parent an opportunity to be positive. Consequently, the clinician models and trains the parent to incorporate reinforcement for stutter-free speech in the treatment program as often as possible. Recall the comment of Bellack and Hersen that most people find it easier to apply punishment than to learn how to identify a desirable response and reinforce that response. It is necessary to spend much clinical time in training parents to apply verbal and tangible rewards for stutter-free speech. Then, when the time comes to train parents in verbal punishment of stuttering, important steps have been taken toward preventing the parent becoming punitive with the child.

In treatments for young children the required length of stutter-free speech is not measured with precision in the way that occurs with programmed treatments that are described in later sections. Examples of periods of speech that can be required to be stutter-free as a treatment target are "five minutes," "talking about a page in a book," "an utterance," "naming a picture" and "a phone call to grandfather." Often at the start of a treatment program, the clinician will prescribe a goal of stutter-free single-syllable utterances in treatment sessions. Even if the child does not actually require training at this level, such a treatment goal can provide confidence for the child.

Parents frequently expect inappropriate periods of stutter-free speech. There is no point, for example, in requiring the child to produce five minutes of stutter-free speech when the child is incapable of speaking for one sentence without stuttering. Continual assessment of the child is needed to ensure that the most suitable speech duration is selected for reward. If the task is too easy or too difficult, the child will learn nothing. More importantly, if the task is too difficult, the child is likely to become negative about the procedure because of constant failure.

---

[1] It is often argued that the words "stutter" and "stuttering" have a potentially stigmatizing effect.

## Stuttering

As stated already, direct punishment of stuttered speech needs to be done carefully with young children. There is a great deal of scope for things to go wrong due to a child reacting adversely to the negative input. Any parent will attest to the effects of unremitting negative input to a young child, and the same thing will happen if the child feels "nagged" about stuttered speech. Above all else, the child's treatment program needs to be a supportive and positive one in which stutter-free speech can be learned. That goal cannot be realized with excessive negative input.

A little thought from the perspective of a 2- or 3-year-old child is useful. More often than not, at the time of the consultation parents have not directly drawn attention to the child's stuttering. If after the initial consultation the parents suddenly begin to draw attention to stuttered speech, this is likely to be disorienting and upsetting for the child. Most clinicians find that the best way to introduce feedback for stuttered speech is in an extremely graduated fashion, with the first corrections for stuttered speech introduced at a rate of only once or twice each day. During this time, considerable positive feedback to the child is provided, as described above.

## Self monitoring and self evaluation

It is a simple matter to provide on-line reward to a child for identifying stutters as they occur. For example, a parent may say "that was good the way you noticed the bumpy word." As is the case for stutter-free speech, self monitoring skills can be trained in a session format or on-line. An example of training self monitoring in a formal session is a game where the child and parent each have a small screen with a number of blocks behind the screen. The child speaks, and the child and parent place a block on a tower behind a small screen when each stuttering occurs. At the end of a talking period a reward is earned if the child's tower is similar to the parent's. A variation of this game is for the parent to talk and sometimes pretend to stutter, and the child's task is to monitor the parent's faked stuttering. How well a child can monitor stuttering on-line is a good index of how well the treatment is going. It is a particularly encouraging sign if a child not only monitors stutterings but sometimes corrects them on-line without prompting from an adult.

A child can be asked to evaluate speech performance and rewarded for correct evaluation. A child may be required, after a period of speech, to state whether or not speech in that period contained stuttering. The duration of the period of speech in such procedures can range between a single-syllable word and several minutes of conversation. This self-evaluation procedure can be conducted in sessions or on-line.

## Generalization and maintenance

As stated in a previous section, generalization of stutter-free speech in preschool children is not thought to be the problem that it is for adults. This applies particularly to the treatment program described here, and one reason for this might be because the treatment is administered within the child's everyday speaking environment. With parents conducting the treatment, there is virtually never a complaint that the child is stutter-free in the clinic but not outside the clinic.

Maintenance begins when the child has generalized satisfactory speech. The clinician in combination with the parents determine when that has occurred. In making that determination, it is useful to incorporate feedback from persons in the child's speaking environment, such as a preschool teacher. Such a person might be consulted to verify the parents' and the clinician's opinion that the child's speech is generally perceived as normal. Considering that many adults are unable to achieve zero stuttering in everyday speaking situations, that goal may not be appropriate for a preschool child, at least in the first part of maintenance.[1] Some clinicians favor maintenance targets that are slightly above zero stuttering, such as below 0.5 or 1.0% SS. On some rare occasions it may be counterproductive to set maintenance criteria at near-zero levels, and a target below 2% SS may be appropriate. One thing to keep in mind is that, even though maintenance performance criteria may be slightly above zero stuttering, parents can still encourage the child to strive for completely stutter-free speech during maintenance. With this in mind, it may be useful to increase the stringency of the maintenance performance criteria some time after maintenance has begun.

---

[1] This statement does not apply to the treatment process, only to therapy outcome. During the treatment process it is important that children are set tasks that require zero stutterings for success.

# An Example of Management of Early Stuttering

## Background

Paul Smith, a 2-year 10-month-old boy was brought to the clinic by his parents. He attended a preschool kindergarten two days per week. Paul's parents reported that stuttering had begun four months previously. They said that they recalled the time of onset clearly, because Paul had normal speech one day and was stuttering quite severely the next. In fact, Ms Smith said she was surprised one morning during breakfast because he "could not get a word out." During the subsequent four months, the Smiths said that the stuttering was episodic, subsiding almost completely for weeks at a time before returning. This cycle occurred twice. The Smiths said that each time these near-remissions occurred they thought that the stuttering would stop, and this was the reason that they had waited so long to seek help. It was reported that Paul sometimes experienced speech blocks which lasted several seconds, and sometimes these were accompanied by grimacing. At times of severe stuttering, Paul reportedly lipped or whispered speech rather than speaking out loud, and the Smiths thought this meant that he did not want to speak because he was afraid of stuttering.

Paul was taken to the family doctor shortly after the first episode of stuttering. However, the signs of stuttering were mild in the doctor's surgery. The parents said that this may have been the reason they were reassured that there was no cause for concern. They were advised to ignore the problem and that it would resolve. The parents recalled being dissatisfied with this advice at the time, because Ms Smith's father had been troubled all his life by severe stuttering, and had been unable to fulfil his career ambitions because of it. Additionally, two of Ms Smith's four brothers have the disorder, as does one of her three nephews.

The Smiths finally contacted the speech clinic directly and made an appointment during a time when Paul was having particular difficulty. They reported that Paul experienced a lengthy block, and then whispered "Mummy, I can't talk." Subsequent to this experience, they did not attempt to help him with his speech because they became alarmed when a friend said that calling attention to stuttering could worsen it.

Paul has a 12-year old sister who has never stuttered. At the time of the assessment Ms Smith was expecting a baby in two months, and ultrasound results indicated a boy.

## Initial speech measures

Prior to the date of the initial consultation, the Smiths were instructed to bring to the clinic two short tape recordings of Paul stuttering, and also to telephone the clinic if it was not possible to obtain such recordings. The clinic visit was postponed initially because Mr Smith telephoned to say that Paul was stuttering only mildly, if at all, that week, and that it had not been possible to obtain a representative recording. On the second appointment the parents brought to the clinic two tape recordings. The clinician rated these recordings in the presence of the parents and measured 11.3 %SS, 87 SPM (326 syllables) on the first and 7.2 %SS, 113 SPM (539 syllables) on the second. Considering these recordings together, there were seven blocks in excess of 2 seconds. Apart from the blocking as described by the Smiths, these recordings revealed part-word repetitions, with sometimes as many as six repetitions of initial syllables of multisyllabic words.

An initial within-clinic rating was made by means of one-way observation facilities and the cooperation of Mr and Ms Smith. Paul was rated while talking with his parents, and stuttered at 5.1 %SS, 124 SPM (547 syllables), showing the same types of stuttering heard on the tape recordings. The grimacing reported by the Smith's was not observed. The clinician felt that this within-clinic measure was not valid because Paul seemed apprehensive of the new surroundings and tended to speak with short utterances.

## Arranging beyond-clinic speech measures

Paul's parents selected seven speaking situations for severity rating. At the second clinic visit two of these situations were changed because of impracticalities that were discovered during the week. Ms Smith regularly brought severity rating scores to the clinic on visits. Two situations that were rated for severity were simultaneously recorded; in the car on the way to preschool and at bedtime. Ms Smith brought SMST measures for these two situations to the clinic each week. Ms Smith required considerable training in collecting these measures, and her scores did not agree satisfactorily with the clinician's scores until the fourth clinic visit. The initial difficulty was that Ms Smith consistently failed to identify stutters. The clinician provided training with the use of Paul's beyond-clinic recordings and with specially recorded tapes containing simulated stuttering. The stutters on these tapes were counted on-line with Ms Smith following the procedure.

## Treatment design

### Treatment sessions

At the first clinic visit it was established that Paul responded well to a structured treatment task that could be performed each day at different times. A response-cost procedure was found to be effective in combination with praise for stutter-free speech. Five-minute sessions were instigated in the home, and Paul was required to respond to a simple picture stimulus with a single stutter-free utterance. Each session began with a bank of 10 tokens, but one of these was forfeited contingent on each stuttering. The tokens remaining at the end of five minutes contributed towards a small set of toys. A total of 20 tokens accumulated by Paul over a period of time could be used to purchase one of these toys. Care was taken to ensure that, in preference to concluding a session with a loss of all tokens, a session was ended prematurely with Paul retaining one token.

The clinician demonstrated this procedure in the clinic at the first visit. After the clinician saw Mr and Ms Smith conducting the procedure, the clinician was prepared to ask the family to attempt it at home. The Smiths were requested to record two of their attempts at these treatment sessions during the week. After listening to the recordings on the second clinic visit, the clinician was satisfied that the procedure was being conducted satisfactorily. However, some feedback was given concerning the need to identify stuttering promptly. Additionally, the clinician noted that the Smiths called attention to Paul's stuttering using similar language to that used when disciplining him. This error was quickly corrected, and

Ms Smith learned to say "stop" contingent on stutters in a non-emotive and supportive manner.

Paul readily participated in this procedure at home. The Smiths were able to learn to vary the stimulus materials and the rewards to maintain interest. A special "good talking badge" was purchased for Paul to wear during treatment sessions. Sessions were omitted on days that Paul was not willing to participate, although such days occurred rarely. Several treatment sessions each week were conducted outside the home, at Paul's grandmother's house and at kindergarten. After two weeks with the procedure Paul was being required by his parents to produce five stutter-free utterances at a time during sessions. The clinician monitored the procedure by observing Ms Smith conduct a session when she visited the clinic each week with Paul, and also by listening to occasional tape recordings of sessions being conducted.

## On-line treatment

In the second week the clinician introduced on-line feedback. Initially, either Mr or Ms Smith selected a different hour each day during which one of them was with Paul and would be able to attend to his speech. Paul pinned on his "good talking badge" during these periods. Practical difficulties resulted in this one hour being separated into two half-hour periods in each day. In the second through to the fourth week, the Smiths only attended to stutter-free utterances during these periods, offering praise for "no stuck words" as appropriate. From the fourth week onwards, when Paul's speech had begun to improve noticeably (see below), the Smiths called attention to most stutters heard during this period and requested Paul to re-attempt the utterances. Occasionally this procedure was accompanied by overcorrection, because Paul seemed to enjoy this approach. Continually during these periods of on-line feedback, the Smiths provided verbal prompts for stutter-free speech.

During the second week through to the fourth week Paul was rewarded with a token at the end of the half-hour periods for cooperating with remedial efforts. From the fourth week to the sixth week, Paul was rewarded with two tokens if a half-hour period was completely free of stuttering. For the seventh week, one half-hour period each day was assessed covertly by either parent, and at the end of the half-hour it was announced to Paul that an assessment had occurred, and he obtained two tokens if no stuttering had occurred. In the eighth week, the assessment procedure was withdrawn and an attempt was made to reward Paul for self-correction of stuttering on-line. However, apparently because of his age, Paul was never able to participate adequately in this procedure although he enjoyed self-monitoring games in treatment sessions where he attempted to count the same number of stutters as his mother during conversations.

## Parent information, counselling, and discussion

Subsequent to the first visit, Ms Smith brought Paul to the clinic for visits without Mr Smith. On the second visit it became apparent that, despite reassurances given at the first visit, Ms Smith was unconvinced that herself and Mr Smith were not to blame for the development of Paul's stuttering. This area required counselling efforts that occupied portions of subsequent sessions. To supplement these efforts, the clinician supplied literature to Mr and Ms Smith which highlighted the physiological nature of stuttering. The suggestion was offered that Ms Smith should seek a second opinion about Paul's stuttering. To the clinician's knowledge, this option was not pursued.

Another focus of discussion was expectations of the speech of a 2-year old child. Towards the end of the series of clinic visits, Ms Smith was assigning severity ratings of around "4" to speech that the clinician judged, on the basis of the two beyond-clinic recordings each week, to be perfectly normal. After discussion, it emerged that Ms Smith's ratings were being influenced by pauses and phrase revisions that the clinician considered to be normal speech events. The clinician indicated to Ms Smith what appropriate ratings for the beyond-clinic recordings might be, and a tape recording containing examples of normal 2-year-old speech was played and discussed with her (the clinician had available such a tape, which was constructed for this specific purpose). Additionally, the clinician (with Ms Smith's permission) played a segment of one of the beyond-clinic recordings of Paul to non-clinician staff associated with the clinic. These listeners were asked to indicate whether there was "anything wrong" with the speech on the recordings. All four listeners confirmed that Paul's speech showed no speech or language disorder.

The clinician gave some information about the baby that Ms Smith was expecting. Taking care not to alarm the Smiths, it was explained that this child might be at some risk of stuttering. Although this risk was small, the clinician felt that there might be benefit in discussing appropriate ways of responding should any signs of the disorder appear. It was decided that, should this occur, the Smiths should contact the clinic and they would be given a priority appointment. In this context, the clinician again stressed to the Smiths that stuttering is not caused by parental behavior. The clinician explained that the skills Ms Smith had learned in monitoring Paul's speech would be invaluable in ensuring that any appearance of stuttering in the second child would be detected immediately. The clinician also stressed that, in the unlikely event of the second child requiring treatment, the combination of early intervention and the management skills Ms Smith had learned with Paul would make for an extremely favorable prognosis.

## Clinical progress

Ms Smith and Paul attended the clinic on nine consecutive occasions before maintenance began. After the fourth clinic visit the clinician decided that the Smiths should cease the treatment sessions at home, because they no longer seemed necessary for satisfactory clinical progress. Figure 3 shows the clinician's graph of the various speech measures used during management. Ms Smith's average severity ratings for each week appear on this graph, as do the two beyond-clinic measures each week and the one within-clinic measure each week. The severity ratings appear to be valid because they reflect the same trend as the beyond-clinic SMST scores. These measures all show progressive reductions in stuttering. At around week five, Paul's kindergarten teacher and one of Mr Smith's friends made unsolicited comments that his speech was improving. At week six of management, Paul stuttered rarely.

## Maintenance

At week 10 of management, the clinician and Ms Smith decided to begin maintenance. The following criteria were devised:

1. Mean severity rating less than or equal to 2.0.
2. Zero % SS during a 10-minute telephone conversation with the clinician.
3. Zero SMST in two beyond-clinic recordings.

In order to pass a maintenance assessment, Paul was required to meet these criteria for the week preceding the assessment. The maintenance program was devised so that Paul never attended the clinic, but spoke to the clinician by telephone at some time during the week prior to the assessment. Paul did not know in advance when the clinician would call, and the call occurred at a different day and time for each maintenance assessment. The program was performance contingent, and similar to the schedule presented on page 62, except that Mr or Ms Smith was required to attend the clinic only on M3 and M6. Additionally, an M9 assessment occurred, 32 weeks subsequent to M8. On assessments that Ms Smith did not attend the clinic, she telephoned the clinician and presented the speech measures. On the M3 and M6 assessments, the clinician listened to Ms Smith's recordings of Paul to verify that the SMST criteria had been met.

Paul had little difficulty passing through this program, and regressed to M1 only once. The covert on-line reward system was systematically withdrawn once the maintenance program began. This was done by administering the procedure six days in the first week, five days in the second week, four days in the third week, and so on. This withdrawal occurred without incident. However Mr and Ms Smith decided, on advice from the clinician, to apply the procedure on one randomly-chosen day each week, for a period of six months.

FIGURE THREE: Speech measures for Paul over a 10-week period.[1] Note that the clinician graphed three sets of different data measures with two vertical axes, meaning that one axis is used for two sets of data.

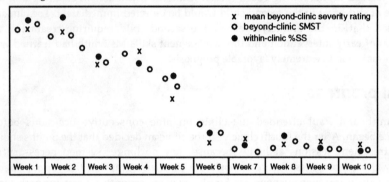

---

[1] This graph is schematic. It is convenient to record each individual daily severity score, not the weekly means as shown in this graph. Daily severity scores are an important source of information about the client's speech performance beyond the clinic.

# Part Four:

# Management of Advanced Stuttering

# Management Phases With Advanced Stuttering

"Advanced stuttering" refers to an adolescent or adult who has been stuttering since the preschool years. The following sections pertain to operant and prolonged speech treatments for advanced stuttering which incorporate either programmed or nonprogrammed instruction. In comparison to early stuttering, more cases of advanced stuttering require programmed instruction, and more cases require formal procedures for generalization and maintenance. Because of this it is useful to think of the management process in various stages. These stages of client management are discussed below, but they are not necessarily discrete. In fact, they overlap, and it would be a mistake to complete one stage before giving any thought to the next. The most effective way of taking a client through treatment is to lay the groundwork for subsequent phases of management. How this can be achieved is indicated below.[1]

## The Preliminary Phase

This is where clients/parents are prepared for the start of treatment and the clinician carefully studies the client's disorder. It is probably the most important management phase because skills are taught to clients and parents that are essential to successful treatment. Procedures to collect within- and beyond-clinic speech measures are established. Parents are taught to supply beyond-clinic measures and the reliability of their measures is established. Older children can supply speech measures for the clinician independently of parents. Adult clients are taught to collect measures of their own speech. The clinician may choose to incorporate some covert speech measures into the management plan, and regular checks determine whether overt measures resemble covert measures.

Perhaps the most important part of the Preliminary Phase is the informing of clients/parents about their eventual responsibility for the effectiveness of the treatment program, because they need to contribute considerable effort in order to achieve durable, stutter-free speech. Effective treatment of advanced stuttering involves substantive lifestyle change, and one of the serious problems that confront clinicians is that it may become apparent well into the management process that a client is not really prepared to make that change. It is critical for the clinician to initially explain the considerable requirements of treatment, and to utilize whatever measures are necessary to determine whether clients are prepared to undertake those requirements. Extensive discussions with clients/parents may be needed to make that determination.

Speech measures are used to establish a baserate of stuttering severity over a period of several weeks, and the clinician uses that baserate to obtain an accurate impression of the client's disorder as well as indices of speech performance against which subsequent improvements can be detected. Treatment procedures do not commence during this period.

---

[1] The outlines of treatments for advanced stuttering presented in Part Four are intended to be neither detailed manuals of clinical procedures nor aids to clinical instruction.

However, it is important to recognize that intervention is not withheld for the sake of obtaining baseline trends: The Preliminary Phase of management is used for training clients/parents in measurement procedures and for whatever information provision, discussion, or counselling is necessary as a prelude to treatment. If those things are not done, it is virtually pointless to proceed with a treatment program.

Another function of the Preliminary Phase is to establish a suitable treatment for the client. Four guidelines to consider in the selection of a treatment are as follows:

1. The response of the client to treatments. The client is trialed with a number of treatments to assess their potential suitability. In particular, the clinician pays attention to the potential efficacy of a variety of operant-based procedures that do not incorporate prolonged speech. This is a particularly important investigation with younger clients. Abbreviated components of different treatments are administered in the clinic in the hope of establishing if one shows promise of controlling the client's stuttering.
2. Preference is given to suitable operant treatments because those treatments are generally easier and quicker to administer and are free of the problems associated with prolonged speech (those problems are discussed in Part Six).
3. The client's willingness to participate in a particular treatment. This is an important consideration because of the arduous nature of many treatments for stuttering and the demands that those treatments place on clients and their families. In addition to exposing the client briefly to the treatment, the clinician needs to ensure that the client is adequately informed about precisely what demands are associated with that particular treatment. This concern is particularly relevant to children. Clinical problems can arise from situations where parents wish a child to undergo treatment but the child does not wish to participate.
4. The final consideration in choosing a treatment is the most important to some clinicians. A treatment which has empirical evidence for its effectiveness inspires more confidence than one which does not. In other words, if there is evidence from clinical trials that a treatment is effective, then that treatment would be preferable to one which has not been researched.

# The Instatement Phase

This is when clients learn to produce stutter-free speech to a criterion level within the clinic. The focus of the Instatement Phase is to find an effective treatment; it is by no means certain that the first treatment selected will be successful. This process of treatment evaluation can be quite time consuming.[1] However, it is worth noting that an effective

---

[1] If the client visits the clinic several times, each week, rather than just once, the process of finding an effective treatment can be completed in a shorter time. Sometimes it is a worthwhile strategy for the client to visit the clinic several times each week during the Instatement Phase of management, and subsequently visit only once per week during the Generalization and Maintenance Phases.

treatment, once completed, should have the capacity to control stuttering for a lifetime. It is also worth noting that if a client is managed for a considerable period of time without establishing an effective treatment, then it is necessary to be able to demonstrate that the clinical time was put to good purpose. Speech performance measures can contribute here by documenting the lack of response of the client to early treatments and the eventual positive response of the client to the final treatment that was chosen.

Towards the end of the Instatement Phase, client/parent contribution needs to be maximized. In the case of children, there is no way a clinician can expect a treatment to be successful without the contribution of skilled parental support. In the case of adults and adolescents, it is the client who must assume the ultimate responsibility for rehabilitation, and most of that responsibility should be assumed by the end of the Instatement Phase. A clinician can only guide a client in eliminating stuttering; it is the responsibility of the client/parents to complete the substantial amount of work that is required to achieve this goal. What can sometimes happen during this phase is that the clinician, inadvertently and gradually, assumes dominant responsibility for the conduct of treatment.

Progress through the Instatement Phase is determined by attainment of treatment session goals. Generalization to beyond-clinic speech situations may occur, but success in treatment sessions is not dependent on this. This is an important point. Generalization need not occur during the Instatement Phase. Of course, steps ought to be taken to increase the possibility that generalization will occur, as discussed in Part Two. But clients or their parents often complain during the Instatement Phase that generalization is not occurring. In which case, the clinician needs to make it clear that this is not the intention of this part of treatment.

At the conclusion of the Instatement Phase it becomes clear what the client's criteria for satisfactory speech should be. Those criteria are described using the speech measures outlined in Part Two. Establishing speech criteria performance is the focus of a behaviorally-based treatment for stuttering, because those criteria determine the clients progression through the critical Generalization and Maintenance Phases which are to follow. This is not meant to suggest that speech criteria established during instatement are inflexible. On the contrary, they are often changed later in the treatment process. But establishing an initial set of performance criteria is a key component of the Instatement Phase of management.

## The Generalization Phase

In this phase systematic procedures are applied to facilitate generalization of newly-learned speech skills. It concludes when the client uses stutter-free speech in situations that are representative of everyday life. Many published treatment programs contain a phase of treatment referred to as "transfer." As mentioned in Part One, "transfer" really refers to a specific technique—sequential modification—which may be used to achieve generalization. Successful treatment programs are generally the result of a variety of techniques applied to enhance generalization. To routinely progress clients through a program of sequential modification, without regard to any other procedure for generalization, would limit the value of a treatment program.

It may also be problematic if an abrupt boundary is set up between the Instatement and Generalization Phases. The two are combined to some extent for best results. For example, toward the end of the Instatement Phase when the client has made considerable inroads into being able to produce stutter-free speech in the clinic, generalization procedures can be initiated. Perhaps the clinician would begin to shift some of the instatement activities into the client's everyday speaking situations ("train sufficient exemplars"; see Part One). This is preferable to waiting until the client has completed the Instatement Phase before beginning generalization activities.

At the end of the Instatement Phase, the extent of unplanned generalization is assessed, and the necessity for programmed generalization is determined. Some younger children show complete generalization of stutter-free speech and do not require any planned generalization activities. Some clients show partial unplanned generalization, which is often associated with comments such as "my speech is sometimes OK but not always." Some clients show no generalization at all, and they present the greatest clinical challenge during the Generalization Phase. In cases where clients do not achieve any unplanned generalization, it may be useful to implement a sequential modification procedure (see Part One).

## The Maintenance Phase

The Maintenance Phase is where the clinician systematically assists clients/parents to ensure that treatment gains are durable. The purposes of maintenance and procedures to manage it are discussed in Part One. A study by Ingham ( 1981a) demonstrates that self-evaluation training may assist clients with long-term maintenance of stutter-free speech. Ingham (1987) presents a model of how self-evaluation trials may be used as a "lead in" to the Maintenance Phase; the client tape records beyond-clinic speech performance and evaluates those recordings. In Ingham's (1987) model, the client must succeed in six, consecutive, weekly self evaluation (SE) assessments before being admitted to the Maintenance Phase. This means that the client may only enter the Maintenance Phase of management when adequate self evaluation skills have been demonstrated.

If self-evaluation skills are established during the Instatement Phase, then it is wise to include them in maintenance activities. Ingham (1987a) outlines a procedure where clients/parents evaluate their performance and determine whether they should progress to the next step or regress to step one; in other words, a self-managed maintenance program. With this procedure, the client/parents are prescribed only one or two clinic visits during the Maintenance Phase. At steps that do not involve a clinic visit, the family telephones the clinician to report the outcome of each step. If this client/parent managed program is unsuccessful, it may then be changed to include clinic visits at each step. But the benefits of a self-managed maintenance program are that it requires less clinical time and that the responsibilities of clients/parents are increased.

# Preventing Relapse With Advanced Stuttering

The extensive problem of posttreatment relapse with advanced stuttering might suggest that the disorder is innately intractable. Regardless of whether that is true or not, it is still the clinician's responsibility to do all that is possible to prevent relapse. The best clinical approach is to foresee relapse and take steps to prevent it. Building systematic maintenance activities into treatment is one way that this can be done. The following sections mention other ways that treatment can be designed with foresight about preventing relapse.

## Make sure that there will be sufficient gains from the treatment

Most people would rather not stutter. However, maintenance of stutter-free speech requires a lot of work from clients, and there is no guarantee for every client that the work will be worth it. Some clients do not gain many benefits from acquiring stutter-free speech; their lives do not change in a major way when they cease to stutter. Under those circumstances it is not surprising that relapse might occur. It is important before treatment for the clinician to obtain some idea of the gains that a client expects from treatment. Often clients have unrealistic expectations of how their lives will change when they acquire the capacity to speak without stuttering. In which case, it is the responsibility of the client to provide a realistic appraisal of the gains that might accrue from stutter-free speech.

## Make sure that the client really wants the treatment

It is worth reiterating that treatments discussed here are those concerned with the elimination of stuttered speech. It would cause problems if a client received such a treatment when that was not really what the client wanted. As noted previously, there is little point in treating clients for conditions about which they do not complain. Most clients do complain about stuttered speech (Andews, 1984b), but many do not. So it may be incautious to assume that a client's complaint is about stuttered speech. Other complaints may be about speech anxiety, or being unable to cope with the disorder, or of lack of information about the disorder, or lack of support. In such cases it may, or it may not, be appropriate to eliminate stuttered speech. It can occur that a client believes that stuttering is the cause of various personal problems. Serious emotional problems can cause people to make misjudgments, and someone with such problems can believe that they arise from stuttered speech. In some cases, stuttered speech is among the least of a person's problems.

## Make sure the client is sufficiently motivated for the treatment

Relapse to stuttered speech can occur simply because clients/parents are unwilling to do what is required to sustain stutter-free speech in the long run. Certainly, all clients require counselling at some part of the Maintenance Phase of treatment in order to maintain their enthusiasm. Nonetheless, provision of information before the treatment is an effective way to prepare clients for what is required of them during maintenance. It is also effective in screening out clients who are not really prepared to commit themselves to treatment. Perhaps even more effective in identifying insufficiently motivated clients is the procedure described in Part Two, where motivation itself is managed as a desirable client response.

## Make sure that the client knows what to expect as an outcome of treatment

It is always easy to tell clients about the positive aspects of completing a successful treatment. For example, a clinician might tell a client that a treatment could establish stutter-free speech, that socializing could be easier, that career prospects could improve, and that self confidence could increase. However, it would be unrealistic to overlook some of the negative features of a successful treatment. For example, a clinician may tell a client that regular speech practice will be necessary for the rest of life, and that short periods of relapse may be expected from time to time with accompanying feelings of despondency. If a client is not informed that such things may occur, and they do occur, they may be sufficiently demoralizing to undermine the maintenance of stutter-free speech.[1]

---

[1] Those who are considering undertaking treatment for stuttering can obtain an perspective on such things by talking to treated clients.

# Nonprogrammed
# Operant Treatment

## Punishment

Research considered in Part Five suggests that punishment is the most effective of the operant techniques which reduce stuttering. However, such procedures are not suitable for all clients. In fact, many clients, especially children, dislike them and do not wish them to be part of their treatment. So, during the Preliminary Phase of management when treatments are tested for their suitability, it is important to determine whether punishment should be excluded from a client's treatment.

### Time-out (TO)

The basic procedure of TO is for the clinician to converse with the client and, contingent on stuttering, to say "stop" and break eye contact for a short interval, after which the conversation is resumed. A few seconds is sufficient for a TO interval—the duration of the interval appears not to be crucial. Because the procedure is intrinsically aversive, the clinician needs to supplement it with support and encouragement during and at the conclusion of each trial. Costello (1975) presents case reports of a TO treatment.

Time-out has some striking advantages as a treatment. First, it can be adapted for younger clients. One creative way of doing this was demonstrated by (Martin, Kuhl & Haroldson (1972), who used a puppet, rather than a person, to present the TO stimulus to children.[1] The creative clinical use of a puppet serves effectively to remove the human component from the procedure; it is not the clinician but the puppet who presents the TO stimulus. Second, an extremely useful thing about TO is that clients can administer it to themselves in everyday speaking situations. They can "time themselves out," and this is a good way to "mediate generalization" (see Part Two). As is the case with any operant treatment for stuttering, it can be a good idea to combine TO with token reinforcements if it is used with children, and to vary the reinforcement schedule systematically.

Treatment sessions during the Instatement Phase use an "ABA" format, where "A" is a period of conversation with the clinician and "B" is a set of treatment trials. Each session begins with a number of A conditions, followed by a number of treatment (B) trials, followed again by a number of A conditions. The purpose of this ABA format is to establish, and to reaffirm in each session, the capacity of the TO procedure to control stuttering. Further, the final A condition establishes whether treatment effects generalize into adjacent speaking situations. Costello's (1975) treatment records show how the instatement program ends when the client can maintain stutter-free speech without the TO procedure. Speech measures can be graphed on-line during each session.

Each trial might be from 200 to 500 syllables, depending on the speech rate of the client. Around 2-3 minutes per trial is desirable. If the length of each trial is held constant, there is

---

[1] The subjects in that experiment were younger than 5 years. Clinical use of the technique may not be suitable for children that young.

no need to calculate %SS and SPM because it is sufficient merely to graph the number of stutters and the time taken to speak the syllables during each trial. A record of the time taken to speak the syllables in each trial is essential to ensure that the treatment is not, in effect, rate control. The reason for this is that a client may respond to the procedure by reducing speech rate, which probably will reduce stuttering (see Part One). Unless a record of syllables spoken per clinical trial is made, a clinician may be convinced that the TO is controlling stuttering when, in reality, stuttering is controlled by reduced speech rate. An alternative approach is to base the clinical trials on time spent talking. For example, each trial could be 2 minutes of cumulative speaking time.

The program is conducted with TO trials until satisfactory results are obtained during clinic sessions. When the client succeeds with monologue, treatment trials can involve conversation. Final treatment trials might involve a self-evaluation procedure that incorporates self-imposed TO. In other words, the client is required to self-impose time out in order to pass a trial. This makes good sense if the clinician plans that the client will learn to self-impose TO in everyday situations as part of the treatment.

FIGURE FOUR. Some preliminary treatment sessions from the Instatement Phase of a client's treatment with a TO treatment program. See text for discussion.

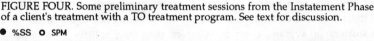

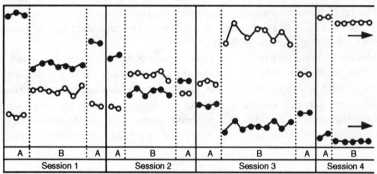

Figure 4 shows the clinical course of the Instatement Phase of a TO treatment program conducted within the clinic. Each trial consists of 3 minutes of cumulative speaking time. The SPM scores increase with the decreasing %SS scores, which verifies that the client is not eliminating stuttering merely by reducing speech rate. After several more sessions than are shown in Figure 4, the client normally is able to show a "flat graph." In other words, the client is able to produce near-zero stutters in A and B conditions. At which time the clinician may change the type of speech which is the basis of the trials. For example, if the data in Figure 4 were from monologue, then the clinician may choose to redo the treatment trials with a conversational speech format.

## Response cost

Response cost is another way of using punishment in treatment. It can be useful with children who will not tolerate TO, because it does not involve direct negative stimulation. Tokens are the most effective materials for response cost. The child receives a bank of tokens at the start of the session and loses one contingent on stuttering. The child retains the tokens remaining at the end of a trial, or a set of trials. The tokens may be exchanged for tangible items. It is important for the clinician to be careful to modify punishing schedules so that the client's bank of tokens is not depleted at the end of a treatment session. The question should not be whether the child will have any tokens remaining at the end of the session, but how many tokens the child will have. Response-cost procedures can be combined with reinforcement procedures, such as those described below. In such a format, the child can recover lost tokens by producing periods of stutter-free speech.[1]

# Reinforcement

One advantage of rewarding clients for criterion segments of stutter-free speech is that it is a positive and supportive thing to do. Shaw and Shrum (1972) demonstrate one possible way that this can be done. The treatment format is organized in the same way as TO described above, except for the contingency arrangements. As the client speaks in monologue or conversation (whichever the treatment task might be), periods of stutter-free speech of the required interval are rewarded with tokens and/or praise. Of course, it is not essential to use tokens, but they are particularly convenient in this context, especially when children are involved.

As with TO, the required period of stutter-free speech can be prescribed in terms of a number of syllables or a period of time. A target number of stutter-free syllables for treatment trials is calculated taking into account the stuttering rate of the client. For example, if a client stutters, on average, every 50 syllables, then there is little point in prescribing a treatment target of 10 stutter-free syllables (unless the point of such a task is for the client to gain some confidence). A target number of syllables can be calculated that will result in an optimal error rate for satisfactory treatment.[2]

Syllables are counted on-line, but the counter is zeroed when stuttering occurs. A token is earned when the target number of syllables or time is reached. The recommended number of syllables per trial, and the ABA treatment session format, are the same as described above for TO. Measures graphed are the number of stutter-free units of the target number of syllables during each trial. The change from monologue to conversation, and the introduction of self-evaluation trials, can also occur in the manner specified previously for TO.

# Shaping

Shaping is a procedure where a desired behavior is acquired in steps, where each step is more similar to the desired behavior. In the case of stuttering, treatments can shape stutter-free speech. A later section describes ways to do this using programmed instruction. Those treatments prescribe speech practice at predetermined durations of stutter-free speech which are systematically increased. However, this programmed instruction approach to shaping stutter-free speech may not be necessary. One way of ensuring that the client achieves stutter-free speech practice at the optimum level might be simply to require the client to attempt to increase the duration of stutter-free speech achieved in a previous clinical trial. Having a client improve an existing performance level, rather than attempting to meet predetermined performance levels, might be a a more logical way of shaping stutter-free speech.

---

[1] There have been attempts to base adult intensive treatment programs on token enconomies, where tokens are earned and used to purchase necessities and luxuries in a residential setting.

[2] Note that the target number of stutter-free syllables is not systematically increased in this program. To do so would be an example of programmed instruction, which is considered in a subsequent section.

Some hypothetical results of such a treatment program are shown in Figure 5. A treatment session consists of the client's attempts to increase the previous duration of stutter-free speech attempted. Measures are minutes and seconds of stutter-free speech. In the example in Figure 5, the clinician has recorded only the client's successful attempts, and noted how many trials on each occasion were required to increase the duration of stutter-free speech from the previous target. As with the TO program, the clinician has measured speech rate to ensure that the client has not merely spoken slower in order to increase the durations of stutter-free speech. With young children, tokens might be a useful addition to this program.[1] The program target might be 5 minutes of monologue, followed by a repeat of the program with conversational targets. A third stage of the program might then incorporate self evaluation, where the client conducts the program and is corrected if an error occurs in detecting stuttering.

FIGURE FIVE: Some preliminary treatment sessions from the Instatement Phase of a client's treatment with a nonprogrammed shaping procedure. See text for explanation. Solid data points represent durations of stutter-free speech achieved in each clinical trial, and the open data points represent speech rate at each clinical trial. The numbers recorded below the data points represent the number of attempts required for the client to improve on the duration of stutter-free speech in the previous trial.

● %SS    O SPM

| 1 3 5 1 3 1 7 28 29 | 2 34 1 33 7 1 9 2 6 | 2 2 4 7 4 7 7 9 9 2 8 3 | 3 2 5 1 7 8 |
|---|---|---|---|
| Session 1 | Session 2 | Session 3 | Session 4 |

---

[1] For young children, one clear advantage of this program over TO is that it is logistically far easier to manage at home and also requires parents to have fewer clinical skills. Time-out may seem like a simple thing to do, but it requires a surprising amount of skill, especially with children. Another advantage of this procedure for children is that it contains fewer aversive stimuli. Also, many children enjoy seeing the graph of their performance rise, as in Figure 5, and they can be involved in constructing it.

# Programmed Operant Treatment

## Example of a GILCU program

The previous section demonstrated how stutter-free speech may be shaped with nonprogrammed instruction. If it is considered to be necessary, there are several published programmes for using programmed instruction to shape stutter-free speech. Ryan (1974) is generally credited with the first such published procedure. It is known as gradual increase in length and complexity of utterance (GILCU). Costello's (1983) program is one of several variations on this technique (for example, Johnson, Coleman & Rasmussen, 1978; Mowrer, 1975). Costello (1984) reported that 33 clinical hours were required for the completion of the program with an 11-year-old client. This information might be of value in determining whether a client's rate of progress is satisfactory.

The ELU program incorporates principles of shaping, plus verbal and tangible reinforcement and punishment. The treatment target is gradually increased from 1 through to 6 stutter-free syllables, then from 3 seconds through to 5 minutes of stutter-free monologue, then from 2 minutes to 5 minutes of stutter-free conversation. The program is for instatement only, with programmed generalization procedures introduced as necessary when the client reaches the 5-minute conversation target.

Steps 1-6 of the treatment require the client to produce from 1- to 6 syllable stutter-free utterances. Sets of stimulus cards are used to elicit these utterances. After Step 6 the client is required to produce longer and longer intervals of stutter-free speech. If necessary, the clinician introduces "additives" to assist with control of stuttering. Costello recommends "gentle onsets" and/or rate control as needed. "Gentle onsets" is a term used to describe one of the components of prolonged speech, which will be discussed in a later section. When a stutter-free 5-minute monologue is achieved (Step 16), the following target is a 2-minute conversation. Until this point where a conversational response is required, pauses in speech are considered error responses, whether they are stutters or difficulties in thinking of things to say. At Step 19 (4-minute conversation) the client is not stopped when stuttering occurs, but is informed at the end of the trial if stuttering occurred. Correct and incorrect responses to each clinical trial are scored, and at the completion of each step the percentage of correct responses and the number of responses to meet criterion are recorded.

There are 20 steps in this program, but this number is rarely sufficient, because "branching steps" are required. Costello's (1984) report shows how branching steps can be used. They are intermediate steps for use when the client fails to make a transition from one program step to the next. For example, if a client cannot manage the transition from 10 to 20 seconds of stutter-free monologue, the clinician may introduce a step involving a 15-second target. As with any speech training, a high client success rate is maintained, and Costello's (1984) case report shows how this can be achieved with the use of branching steps.

Backup reinforcers are exchanged for tokens in the program.[1] Praise is used with a 1:1 fixed ratio, but the tokens are administered in 1:1, 2:1, 3:1 ratios as the program progresses. The exchange rate for tokens is varied through 10:1, 25:1, 50:1 as the program progresses, but are altered at the clinician's discretion to maximize the child's enthusiasm. A trial ceases contingent on stuttering and the word "stop," so in effect the program incorporates a TO stimulus.

Treatment targets vary throughout the program, and are expressed as the number of consecutive, stutter-free trials that the client must achieve. For example, at Step 3 (stutter-free, 3-syllable utterance), the client is required to achieve 10 consecutive successful trials to progress to Step 4 (stutter-free 4-syllable utterance). Fail criteria also vary throughout the program, and are expressed as the total numbers of trials that may be attempted without success. In other words, clients may attempt only a certain number of trials without meeting the applicable criterion. At Step 3, for example, the client is permitted only seven consecutive failures before a branching step is introduced.

# Programmed operant treatment: Final comments

Programmed operant treatments may be ideal starting points in a search for an effective treatment for early stuttering, because they can be used as a basis for prolonged-speech treatment if necessary. In the ELU program, for example, Costello describes how features of prolonged speech can be introduced into the ELU treatment. The procedure provides the clinician with a treatment where it is not necessary to decide a priori whether a certain client should have programmed instruction in simple or complex treatments. If there is some doubt, establishment procedures can begin with the ELU program without modification. If progress is satisfactory, then modifications are unnecessary. However, if the clinician finds that progress is unsatisfactory, then the features of prolonged speech can be incorporated into treatment trials.

It is worth noting that published methods of programmed operant treatment are not necessarily in the best interest of every client. A treatment might be made more suitable for a client if the clinician explores creative ways to apply it. One such variation might involve the ELU program. For example, every client may not need to begin that program at the 1-syllable level. Some people who stutter mildly may be able to begin the program at a much later stage. With this in mind, a clinician could assess a client before treatment to determine a starting point for the program. A client who stutters on average once every 30 seconds might begin a treatment based on ELU at a treatment target of 40 seconds of stutter-free speech.

In order to administer an operant treatment with programmed instruction, it is not necessarily best to adapt existing programs such as in the example given above. With a little clinical creativity, it is possible to devise a number of novel programs. For example, consider the nonprogrammed time-out treatment described on pages 92-93 and depicted in Figure 4. With the use of clinical procedures based on a changing criterion experimental design (Barlow & Hersen, 1984), it is possible to program a time-out treatment by requiring the client to systematically reduce stuttering according to gradually reducing targets of %SS during clinical trials. A treatment session from such a programmed approach to time-out treatment would somewhat resemble that depicted in Figure 5 on page 95.

---

[1] Costello (1993) presents a checksheet which is used to select backup reinforcers which would be suitable for a child, and a set of guidelines for administering the token reinforcement system.

# Programmed Prolonged Speech

## Introduction

Prolonged speech is not a new technique for the control of stuttering. Borman (1969) cites the writing of an 18th century physician that describes a speech pattern which seems similar to those in use today. In the latter half of this century, prolonged-speech treatments underwent systematic research and development which led to their current popularity. Goldiamond's (1965) experiments were the start of those modern developments (see Part Two).

There are many modern variants of prolonged speech. Although these treatments have different labels (for example "smooth speech" and "precision fluency shaping"), Ingham (1984) points out that it is futile to consider whether there are relevant differences between these variations of the procedure. One reason for this is that there is no operational definition for any of these speech patterns. Another reason is that they probably are more similar than different; it is likely that they function in the same way to control stuttering. In learning the speech patterns which control stuttering in these different prolonged speech treatments, clients acquire skills described with terms such as "easy phrase intitiation," "phrase continuity," "continuous vocalization," "continuous airflow," "soft contacts," and "gentle onsets."

The components of programmed prolonged speech treatment can be summarized as follows:

1. Teach clients a speech pattern that can replace stuttered speech.
2. Shape that speech pattern towards speech that sounds natural to the listener and feels normal to the speaker.
3. Systematically instruct clients to use that speech pattern to eliminate stuttering during everyday situations to the extent required.
4. Systematically instruct clients to maintain stutter-free speech for many years

The above sequence is not intended to suggest that this type of treatment consists of discrete steps that should be conducted in a certain order. On the contrary, all these clinical components are conducted more or less concurrently.

## Treatment formats

### Intensive residential

In one application of intensive prolonged-speech treatment, a group of clients lives in the treatment setting for the duration of the program. The specialized nature of the residential format tends to make it a service provision format which only a small number of treatment centres are capable of delivering. Apart from this, major disadvantages of this format are its cost, the practical difficulties it presents for clinicians and clients, and its disruption of the routine of a speech clinic. It also is problematic that clients do all their learning of stutter-free speech outside their customary speaking environments, which probably does not facilitate generalization (see Part Two). An advantage of the format is that clinicians are able to obtain control of, and carefully regulate, the speaking environment of the clients. Intensive residential formats are the most controlled method of replacing stuttered speech with prolonged speech. Because of this they are an ideal "last resort" for clients who have not responded to other treatment efforts.

### Intensive nonresidential

This involves treatment of a group of clients for a substantial number of hours (more than eight) each day over a period of from one to three weeks. Clients return home at the end of each treatment day. The disadvantages of the treatment format are, to a considerable extent, the same as those cited above for the residential format. An advantage of this approach over the residential format is that it bypasses the practical difficulties of residential facilities. However, a major disadvantage is that the benefit of the intensive setting—complete control of clients' speaking environments—is lost when clients return home at night and on weekends. Some examples of intensive prolonged speech treatment programs conducted in Australia are Andrews, Neilson, and Cassar (1987),[1] Ingham (1987), and Manusu, Boycott, Grant, and Khanbhai (1991).

### Nonintensive

Prolonged speech treatment can be administered using customary clinical arrangements, where the client makes one or two visits to the clinic each week, or as many as needed. There are several advantages to this procedure (Onslow & Ingham, 1989), including that it does not disrupt clinical routine. It also allows the client every opportunity to gradually generalize a new speech pattern into daily activities. A disadvantage of the format is the amount of time taken by the client to achieve and generalize stutter-free speech. Although the time in hours of speech practice to reach that goal might be the same, intensive programs allow clients to meet that goal in fewer days. It is sometimes argued that a disadvantage of nonintensive prolonged speech is that the client does not obtain the support of a group of peer clients during treatment.

## Example of a prolonged speech program

This section outlines a program described by Ingham (1987a). There are many similar published programs, and presentation of this one is not intended to suggest that it is the most effective. Nor is there any intention to suggest that a residential intensive program is preferable to an nonresidential intensive program. Most importantly, it is not intended to suggest that intensive formats are the best way to conduct this type of treatment. On the contrary, as noted above, there are reasons to believe that once- or twice-weekly clinic visits are a more desirable way to administer a prolonged speech treatment.

The reason that the Ingham (1987a) program is described here is to provide some details about how programmed instruction can be used to teach clients prolonged speech. The package itself can be adapted as required. For example, it can be adapted for use in a once- or twice-weekly visit format. Also, clinical practice in Australia has shown that clinicians

---

[1] An overview and discussion of this program is presented by Neilson and Andrews (1993).

adapt such programs according to their needs and the needs they perceive their clients have. There can be no doubt that some—or even all—clients will benefit from individually designed aspects of a prolonged speech treatment.

The program consists of four treatment phases, which are outlined in the sections below. The Instatement and Transfer Phases are conducted in the residential setting, and half of the Self-Evaluation Phase and all of the Maintenance Phase are conducted in a nonresidential format.

## The Instatement Phase

In this phase clients learn in six stages to replace stuttered speech with prolonged speech. This process occurs during monologues which are called rating sessions. During rating sessions, clients receive feedback about speech performance after each minute. Learning to speak without stuttering also occurs in group sessions, which are formal meetings for conversation held among clients and clinicians. The purpose of the group sessions is to foster normal conversational speech skills. During the Instatement Phase, then, clients learn the required speech pattern and also learn to use that speech pattern in conversation during group sessions. The Instatement Phase is divided into six stages, each of which is named according to the target behaviors required. These stages are described below.

*Stages 40, 70, 100.* These stages are named according to the speech rate target requirement in each of them: 40 SPM, 70 SPM, and 100 SPM (plus or minus 20 SPM). Another important target behavior in these stages is *zero stuttering* (a target that continues at most times in the program). The terms "continuous vocalization," "soft contacts," and "gentle onsets" refer to target behaviors involved in prolonged speech. These prolonged speech target behaviors are taught by clinicians with the assistance of tape recorded models. Changes in the speech pattern occur across Stages 40, 70, and 100, and this is the start of the shaping process towards natural-sounding speech.

Each stage contains six steps (for example; 70/1, 70/2, 70/3, 70/4, 70/5, 70/6). To pass through a stage, six consecutive steps must be completed with correct target behaviors. Failure at any step results in regression to the first step in that stage. Another failure at that first step means regression to the previous stage. Therefore, a client can progress through to Stage 100 but later be required to return to Stage 70, or even Stage 40. Increasing numbers of syllables are required in rating sessions through these three stages; 300 syllables in Stage 40, 500 in Stage 70, and 700 in Stage 100.

*Stages Na, Nb, Nc.* These stages are conducted in the same manner as the previous three, with the exception that clients may speak at any speech rate they wish. However, an additional target behavior is included: *criterion or below-criterion speech naturalness* is required in addition to zero stuttering. Speech naturalness is measured using the 9-point scale described in Part One, and the clinician scores naturalness and feeds this back to the client during rating sessions after every minute of speech. All rating sessions are 1300 syllables in duration. During these three stages, clients may exaggerate or minimize features of prolonged speech to the extent they wish, providing they remain stutter-free and maintain their target level of speech naturalness.

During Stages Na, Nb and Nc, the naturalness of stutter-free speech is reduced in three steps down to a score of 2 on the naturalness scale, or as close to this level as the individual client can achieve. The naturalness criteria for Stages Na, Nb and Nc are calculated from mean naturalness scores assigned during the last rating session in Stage 100 (100/6). The goal of the program is a naturalness score of 2, so this is subtracted from the mean naturalness score during Stage 100/6. The result is then divided by three to form the naturalness criteria for Na, Nb, and Nc. For example, if the mean naturalness score for Stage 100/6 is 7.0, then 5.0 is divided by three to give 1.7. This value of 1.7 represents the differences in naturalness requirements across Na, Nb, and Nc; the target for Na is 5.3 or below, the target for Nb is 3.7 or below, and the target for Nc is 2.0 or below.

When a client has completed a succession of six stutter-free rating sessions at Stage Na, the clinician calculates the mean naturalness score for those six rating sessions. If this mean naturalness score is equal to or below the Na target naturalness, the client progresses to Stage Nb. If not, the client attempts another sequence of six rating sessions in an attempt to achieve the Na target. Clients are allowed three sets of six rating sessions when attempting to achieve target speech naturalness. Care is taken that this procedure does not pressure clients to achieve target speech naturalness in a short period of time. With some clients there is a trade-off between stuttering and speech naturalness, and it is not possible to achieve optimum naturalness and zero stuttering simultaneously. Such clients may, in fact, improve naturalness scores at some time after the conclusion of the Instatement Phase. However, it is critical to identify those clients who should not attempt to obtain normal levels of speech naturalness during the Instatement Phase.

## The Transfer Phase

In this phase sequential modification is used to attempt to generalize stutter-free, natural-sounding speech. Clients are required to use stutter-free speech in conversation with persons outside the clinic. This is achieved by tape recording themselves in beyond-clinic speaking assignments. Target behaviors for recorded assignments are zero stuttering and speech naturalness equal to or below the target for Nc. The task structure of the Transfer Phase mirrors that of the Instatement Phase. Six 1300-syllable assignments are completed: Male stranger, female stranger, telephone, friends, family, and shopping. Transfer assignments are sequenced the same way as Instatement rating sessions (for example; Shopping/1, Shopping/2, Shopping/3, Shopping/4, Shopping/5, Shopping/6) with the same contingencies for success and failure to meet target behaviors. In the Transfer Phase, the rating sessions of the Instatement Phase do not cease completely. A number of 1300-syllable rating sessions are conducted throughout each day. Failure to meet program targets (zero stuttering and criterion speech naturalness) in these rating sessions means that the previous transfer assignment is failed and, therefore, the client regresses to a preceding transfer task.

## The Self Evaluation Phase

Long-term maintenance is an unrealistic goal if clients are unable to accurately monitor and evaluate their speech, so this Phase prepares the client for maintenance with self evaluation training. Clients are trained to correctly self evaluate. Two components of the Self Evaluation Phase are described bellow.

*The SE I Phase.* This phase is conducted in the residential setting, and overlaps the last portion of the Transfer Phase. The regular 1300-syllable rating sessions become self-evaluation sessions. In the Self-Evaluation Phase rating sessions, the target is not zero stuttering, or target speech naturalness, but correct self-evaluation of those speech dimensions. In other words, the treatment goal changes to self evaluation, and although the client may stutter or exceed the speech naturalness criterion, the client may succeed in the treatment task by identifying that off-target performance.

*The SE II Phase.* For this part of the Self Evaluation Phase the client visits the clinic each week after the residential portions of the program. This is the first time during the program that the client's speech is released from continuous environmental controls. In the residential portions, consequences were attached to any stuttering that clinicians detected outside rating sessions or assignments. Release from this sort of control can cause problems for the clinician during SE II. At each weekly clinic visit the client completes six 1300-syllable within-clinic monologue tasks (three telephone calls and three monologues to a clinician) and presents tape recordings of six 1300-syllable beyond-clinic conversations (two friend, two family, and two telephone). At any part of the SE II Phase, any stuttering or above-target naturalness in a rating session results in failure at that step.

When the SE II Phase is completed satisfactorily, the client progresses into the Maintenance Phase. The SE II phase can require a long time to complete, but it is essential that, before entering the maintenance phase, the client has skills in producing stutter-free speech in everyday situations, and has the capacity to self-evaluate performance in doing so.

## The Maintenance Phase

The basic principle of the Maintenance Phase is described in Part Two; maintenance of program targets is treated as a clinical response. If program requirements are maintained, the client is rewarded with less frequent self-assessment and clinic visits. Beyond-clinic assessments occur in the week preceding each maintenance step. As the client progresses successfully through maintenance, assessments become less frequent. The maintenance schedule is similar to that presented on page 61, with steps occurring at the following number of weeks following completion of SE II: 1, 1, 2, 2, 4, 4, 8, 8, 16, 16, 32, and 32. Failure at any step means returning to the first step, where there is one week to the next maintenance step. The maintenance schedule lasts 126 weeks if the client succeeds at every step, and the last two steps are separated by 32-week intervals.

Clients may regress to the start of the maintenance program on several occasions. As with all programmed instruction, the client probably will not learn anything without failing at one or two clinical tasks. A maintenance program is no exception. The client is learning how to maintain stutter-free speech, and some failed clinical trials are a natural part of that learning process. There are two variants on how this maintenance schedule is administered, which are discussed below.

*Self Managed Performance Contingent Schedule (SMPCS).* In this schedule the client, not the clinician, determines progress through maintenance. Six beyond-clinic recordings are made in the week prior to each step, and the client evaluates these and determines whether the recordings meet program requirements. If the client determines that the tapes meet program requirements, the next maintenance step is attempted after the scheduled number of weeks. If not, the client re-attempts the first maintenance step in the following week. It is recommended that during the SMPCS maintenance procedure the client contacts the clinic each week to report on progress.

At the maintenance steps 10 weeks and 126 weeks after SE II, clients return to the clinic with recordings made to that date. At this clinic visit the client must pass six within-clinic 1300-syllable speaking tasks, and the clinician randomly checks that tapes have been evaluated correctly. Any incorrect evaluation of beyond clinic tapes, or any stuttering or above-criterion speech naturalness in a clinic speaking task means that the client returns to the first step of the maintenance schedule.

*Clinician Managed Performance Contingent Schedule (CMPCS).* If the client fails to progress satisfactorily with a self-managed maintenance procedure, this schedule is used in its place. It is identical except that the client must return with tapes to the clinic at each maintenance step. The tapes are assessed by the clinician, who determines whether they meet program requirements. The clinician also conducts within-clinic speaking tasks at each visit, which the client must pass in order to proceed to the next step.

# Programmed rate control

On some occasions it may be useful to construct a treatment program to help clients control stuttering solely by reducing their rate of speech. Most published prolonged-speech programs include speech rate among performance criteria, so rate control programs can be thought of as an adaptation of prolonged speech. Rate control may be effective if the clinician wishes to enhance the benefits of an operant treatment such as TO or ELU. Ingham and Packman (1977) and Costello (1983) provide examples of how this might be done. Rate control may also be effective for clients with mild stuttering which they wish to control in specific situations. In some cases it may be realistic to consider rate control if assessment shows that rate reduction is useful in controlling a client's stuttering. But if either the client has severe stuttering or requires stuttering to be eliminated in all speaking situations, then probably it is better to consider some other treatment.

The basic procedures in a program of rate control are as follows:

1. Determine a target speech rate range. An adequate speech rate target range should eliminate stuttering to the extent required, and result in speech which sounds and feels acceptable enough for the client to use regularly.
2. Train the client to conform to the target speech rate range.
3. Train the client to use the target speech rate range in everyday situations. This can be accomplished with the usual procedures for generalization outlined in Part Two. Sequential modification is used often in attempts to generalize rate control.

Rate control can be taught by having the client systematically progress through pre-determined target ranges leading up to the final prescribed target range, as occurs in prolonged speech programs. For example, the client could initially be trained to speak without stuttering in the range of 80-100 SPM, followed by 100-120 SPM, 120-140 SPM, and so on. One problem with this is that clients may practice speech at rates which do not contribute anything to their ultimate achievement of the program requirements. Another problem is that little is currently known about how to prescribe a speech rate for a client (see Part Two).

A better approach might be to use an "$AB_1B_2...B_x$" treatment format to incorporate a changing criterion speech rate target, similar to a changing criterion design for single-subject experimentation (Barlow & Hersen, 1984). This procedure has the advantage of allowing the clinician to determine an appropriate rate for the client, rather than having to speculate about what a target rate range should be. Treatment sessions consist of trials of monologue talking periods of a fixed duration (for example, 2 or 3 minutes). Each 15 seconds, speech rate is measured, and these measures are averaged to form a rate for each trial. Note that, during a continuous monologue, the clinician can measure speech rate by simply counting the number of syllables on-line. For example, 40 syllables spoken in 15 seconds is 160 syllables per minute.[1]

After a stable base rate is obtained, the client is targeted for a reduction of this base rate (for example, 10 percent) in subsequent trials. Syllable counts each 15 seconds are fed back, and the client is required to complete a prescribed number of consecutive 1-minute trials within the target range. If the base rate mean is 300 SPM, then the first target might be 270

---

[1] Some software and equipment for counting syllables and stuttering display SPM on-line.

SPM, plus or minus 20 SPM. When the client succeeds at the first target range, then a second target range is specified (for example, another 10 percent reduction). This reduction process continues until a rate is found where the desirable control over stuttering is attained and also where speech sounds and feels acceptably natural. At this point, the client is required to maintain treatment targets for a number of consecutive trials with less frequent feedback; 30 seconds, 60 seconds, and so on, until criterion stuttering and the target rate can be maintained for five minutes. It is also advisable to integrate conversational speech and self evaluation procedures into instatement rate control sessions.

Figure 6 shows an example of the first part of a treatment session. In this session the prescribed speech rate is indicated with horizontal dashed lines. Measures for each minute of speaking time are graphed, although the client received feedback each 15 seconds. Figure 6 shows that the client is achieving some success because as speech rate reduces (open circles) stuttering rate also reduces (closed circles). Later in the session the clinician might establish a speech rate range where stuttering is reduced to a satisfactory level that can be maintained by the client during subsequent treatment conditions. Examples of subsequent treatment conditions that a clinician may choose would be conditions without feedback, or conversation speech trials in place of monologue.

FIGURE SIX: The first trials in a clinic session designed to find a speech rate which will eliminate stuttering. Each trial consists of 1 minute of continuous monologue. Horizontal dotted lines represent target speech rate ranges. "A" trials are baseline. During "B" trials, the client received feedback about speech rate each 15 seconds.

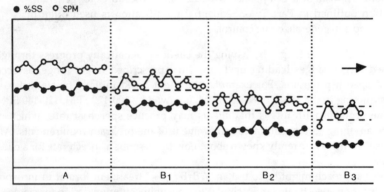

## Programmed prolonged speech: Final comments

There is no reason for clinicians to adhere to the traditional ways that programmed instruction in prolonged speech has been used to eliminate stuttered speech. In fact, that would be an undesirable thing because it would eliminate clinicians' creative efforts and reduce their clinical practices to reiterations of other clinicians' ideas. At many places in this text it has been argued that the value of clinical practice is limited by such reliance on clinical procedures rather than the concepts that underlie them. A striking example of such inflexibility has been clinicians' continued use of the prolonged-speech procedures reported by Goldiamond (1965) to eliminate stuttered speech. In a series of experiments, Goldiamond used programmed instruction to attempt to shape natural sounding, stutter-free speech. Goldiamond's methodology involved (1) establishment of a slow and distorted speech pattern with delayed auditory feedback (DAF), (2) systematic reduction of the DAF level, and (2) systematic increase of speech rate. These also were the salient features of the early prolonged-speech treatment programs, and modern published treatment programs are a direct reflection of this programmed instruction approach to prolonged speech treatment (for example, Andrews, Neilson, & Cassar, 1987; Boberg & Kully, 1985; Ingham, 1987; Shames & Florance, 1980). There have been changes, but all these programs incorporate teaching of an initially slow and distorted prolonged speech, followed by attempts to shape natural sounding speech. This shaping process incorporates clinician instruction about how the speech pattern should change, combined with systematic speech rate increments.

An example of another way of using programmed instruction with prolonged speech is presented by Webster (1980) in an outline of the development of the "Precision Fluency Shaping" program. That outline shows a move away from Goldiamond's treatment model. Instead of the familiar stepwise construction of stutter-free speech at varying speech rates, Webster's current program begins with clients learning the various target behaviors of prolonged speech in single-syllable words. Webster (1980) explains that the rationale for this format is that, in single syllables, the clinician has more opportunity to teach the requisite target speech behaviors that comprise the speech pattern. Although the details are not clear, it is apparent that establishment of stutter-free speech proceeds by means of increments in the duration of speech output, from 2- to 3-syllable words, then to phrases and sentences. Some of these features can be seen in the case history on pages 111-113, where the "GILCU-type" of systematic instruction is applied to prolonged speech. Webster is certainly correct that one advantage of such an approach would be that the clinician is able to closely monitor the way the clients perform targets such as "soft contacts" and "gentle onsets." For example, the clinician might begin the program of instruction by having the client speak a 1-syllable word list using such speech targets. Under such conditions the clinician is able to give precise feedback on the use of "soft contacts" and "gentle onsets" after the utterance of each single syllable. Arguably, in the traditional methods of instruction in prolonged speech, this monitoring of client's performance is not so easy because the treatment tasks involve monologue speech.

There are several issues which concern the traditional ways that clinicians have outlined their procedures in treatment manuals. One such issue is the point at which systematic instruction begins. For example, the treatment program outlined previously begins with a "Stage 40," which is followed by a "Stage 70," then "Stage 100" and so on. But there may be no need for some, or all, clients to begin their program of instruction at "Stage 40." There is certainly no research evidence to indicate which is the best place to start with that—or any other—prolonged speech treatment program. Another issue concerns the use of a "Transfer Phase" in prolonged speech treatment programs, where clients complete tape recorded beyond-clinic speaking assignments. Although some clients may benefit from such a procedure, some may not. Considering the amount of time consumed by formal transfer procedures, it would be a mistake to ignore the possibility that they may not be necessary for some clients.

Perhaps the most dramatic variation of prolonged speech treatment would be to use the procedure without programmed instruction. Certainly, programmed instruction is a useful way of helping clients to achieve skills in a systematic manner (Mowrer, 1982). But this does not mean that programmed instruction is *necessary* for clients to achieve those skills. That seems to be an implication behind the routine incorporation of programmed instruction into intensive programs. Packman, Onslow, and van Doorn (in press) reported the results of a multiple baseline across subjects experiment (Barlow & Herson, 1984) which investigated whether prolonged speech was able to reduce stuttering in laboratory conditions without the programmed instruction that typifies this kind of treatment.

Three adults who stuttered, but who had never received treatment, learned to speak with Stage 40 prolonged speech. Then, subjects practiced Stage 40 prolonged speech for 5 minutes, after which they resumed customary speaking conditions for a 5-minute monologue. In this speaking condition, it was found that all subjects showed clinically significant stuttering reductions, with the stuttering of one subject approaching zero. In a subsequent speaking condition, subjects were informed that prolonged speech is the basis of a treatment procedure, and were instructed to use Stage 40 prolonged speech to eliminate stuttering. All subjects achieved near-zero stuttering rates in this condition, and maintained that effect for a number of speaking sessions. An analysis showed that these stuttering reductions occurred without compromising speech naturalness. The findings of the study are presented graphically in Figure 7.

FIGURE SEVEN: Results from Packman, Onslow, and van Doorn (in press), adapted by permission of the American Speech-Language-Hearing Association. See text for explanation. The solid dots represent %SS scores in five-minute monlogues. Three subjects were studied under three conditions. "A" represents the baseline condition, "B" represents the condition where subjects practiced "Stage 40" prolonged speech before each speaking session, and "C" represents the condition where subjects were told to use the speech pattern to eliminate stuttering.

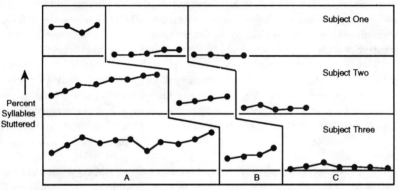

These findings suggest that, for some subjects, systematic instruction in prolonged speech may not be necessary for them to gain benefits from the procedure. In other words, some clients may be able to simply learn prolonged speech skills and then use those skills to produce stutter-free, natural sounding speech, without the need for systematic instruction. Treatment procedures might then concentrate on generalizing those benefits to the extent desired by the client.

# Two Examples of Management of Advanced Stuttering

## Example One:
## Programmed operant treatment

John, an 11-year-old boy, presented initially to the clinic with a stuttering rate of 17.3 %SS (112 SPM) during a 2,000-syllable conversation with the clinician. The routine procedure in the clinic was for parents to bring to the first appointment two beyond-clinic recordings of the child's conversational speech. Prior to the appointment, parents were mailed a set of detailed instructions about how to make the recordings, and in what situations. Parents were also asked to telephone the clinic the day before the appointment to confirm that the recordings had been made. The beyond-clinic recordings which were brought to the clinic at assessment by John's parents showed a similar level of severity to the within-clinic measures. John's speech contained blocks that were often longer than 3 seconds. These long blocks accounted for the low speech rate measured at assessment.

John had never received any treatment, but seemed well motivated to control his stuttering. Therefore the clinician attempted the nonprogrammed operant treatment for early stuttering described in Part Three. This showed no signs of success after a 2-month trial, so John's clinician decided to attempt a programmed operant treatment.

### The initial treatment

The clinician trialed a number of treatments. Unaided self control resulted in no change in stuttering rate. However, the clinician noted that self monitoring with a hand counter—pushed by John contingent on each stuttering—resulted in a 25 percent reduction in stuttering rate. The following assessment trial was a time-out (TO) procedure, and John responded by reducing his stuttering rate by 60 percent. The clinician did not assess any further treatments, deciding that a TO program would be a suitable treatment to attempt initially. One reason for this decision was that John's stuttering decreased a great deal in response to TO at assessment. Further, the clinician favored TO because it allows clients to self-administer the procedure in everyday speaking environments, and John appeared to be the sort of child who would readily participate in such an activity.

The planned management system was outlined in detail to the family. Information was provided about the responsibilities of client and family during management, with special attention to the proposed systematic shift of responsibilities away from the clinician. The clinician pointed out that, as management progressed, John would be making fewer and fewer visits to the clinic as his parents' management skills increased. The clinician took care to ensure that John and his parents understood that there was little point in beginning a course of treatment if their full responsibility for management was not part of the goals of treatment.

John's parents agreed that, for the initial months of intervention, one parent would devote around a 45 minutes each day, excepting Sunday, to the treatment program. It was explained that this time would be devoted to speech measurement procedures and treatment activities. The clinician presented the family with a written presentation of points which were stressed during the assessment, which was a standard procedure in the clinic.

### The Preliminary Phase of treatment

John and his father were scheduled for two clinic visits each week. At the start of each clinic visit the clinician collected %SS and SPM measures during two 2,000-syllable conversations, and recorded them in John's file. One of these conversations was with John and the other conversation was with a relative over the telephone. Once each week, John's father presented measures based on two 10-minute conversations outside the clinic. One of these was John conversing with his brother, and another was conversation at the family dinner table. The latter speech measure was obtained covertly. Each week John's father presented to the clinician SMST measures from these two speaking situations, which he obtained by playing back the tape recordings at another time (see Part Two). All within- and beyond-clinic measures were tabulated and graphed in John's file during the session.

The clinician spent considerable time instructing John's father in basic audio tape recording techniques, and in procedures for eliciting a speech sample. During this time, stable within- and beyond-clinic trends were established.

For the first two weeks of the Preliminary Phase of treatment, the clinician rated beyond-clinic tapes presented by John's father, and devoted much session time to training him in accurate SMST measurement. During the third week of the Preliminary Phase, John's father was able to measure SMST reliably, and the clinician entered these parent scores in the file each session. At this point, the clinician was satisfied that John's father had acquired sufficient skills to support a treatment program. The Preliminary Phase of John's management lasted for four weeks.

### The Instatement Phase of treatment

John's TO treatment program involved nonprogrammed instruction in an ABA format (see Figure 4, page 93). During each session, this procedure promoted changes of from 40-60 percent in John's stuttering severity. However, over a period of five clinic visits John's stuttering rate in the B portion of the sessions showed no sign of approaching zero. Further, no signs were noted of generalized speech improvement into the final A portion of treatment sessions. The clinician also noted that, despite a contract for a substantial tangible reward for the achievement of 5 minutes of stutter-free conversation, John appeared to be losing interest in the procedure because of its essentially negative nature. Considering these factors, the clinician decided to abandon the TO program.

## The second treatment

### The Instatement Phase

The clinician decided that Costello's (1983) programmed ELU shaping procedure (see pages 96-97) would be the next treatment to attempt. John completed the ELU program successfully in 15 weeks and in 23 hours of clinic time. On average, each of the two 1-hour weekly sessions consisted of 15 minutes of within- and beyond-clinic data collection and recording, and 45 minutes of the ELU procedure. The average percentage of correct trials for successful steps was 87 percent, with a range of 65-100 percent. Two branching steps were required, at the 2-minute monologue step and at the 4-minute conversation step.

Despite some training, the clinician was never fully satisfied that John's father would be able to conduct portions of the program at home satisfactorily. Therefore, all steps in the program were conducted by the clinician. However, the clinician was convinced that John's father was able to identify stuttering and give positive feedback appropriately, so John practiced speech trials with his father at home. Those speech trials increased in difficulty according to the progress of the program, but were always slightly easier than the current program requirements. For example, when the ELU program target was 1 minute of stutter-free monologue, John practiced 30 seconds of monologue at home with his father, and when the program target was 5 minutes of conversation, John practiced a 4-minute conversational task at home.

Toward the end of the ELU instatement program, John began to show some generalization of speech skills. This partial generalization was detected by inspection of graphed measures from the two weekly beyond-clinic recordings, and by reports from different people in John's environment who said that his speech had begun to improve. It was decided that less than or equal to 0.5 %SS would be a suitable treatment criterion. This criterion was to apply to tape recordings of John speaking beyond the clinic.

During the Instatement Phase, the clinician used a number of techniques that were designed to increase the chance that any clinic-bound speech improvements would generalize (see Part Two). In addition to his parents, several people gave John positive feedback for periods free of stuttering. These people included his teachers, neighbours and friends (two friends attended clinic sessions at different times). However, the clinician ensured that such people only made general positive remarks about overall speech performance and never offered negative feedback or instruction of any kind. The clinician insisted that only people specifically trained to do so made any comments about stuttered speech. Also, the clinician arranged for some of John's parent-conducted practice sessions to occur when travelling in the family car. The clinician reduced the chance of discriminated learning by ensuring that practice sessions at home occurred far more often than clinic treatment sessions. Additionally, care was taken that home practice sessions occurred in a variety of places within the family home, rather than at the same place on each occasion. Self-monitoring procedures were a prominent component of the latter portions of John's instatement program. John was set a task each day, for a different 1-hour period, to use a hand-held counter to record each stutter that occurred while he was speaking. These 1-hour self monitoring periods included school, home and social situations. The stuttering counts were entered in John's file at each clinic visit.

### The Generalization Phase

During this period of the treatment program, the clinician devised a covert assessment procedure to assist with generalization of treatment gains. Each day, one of John's parents would select a 10-minute period during which his conversation could be monitored covertly. John was aware that such assessments would occur, but was not aware of the time of day that they would occur, or even if one would occur on every day. In fact, the clinician instructed his parents to occasionally miss a day in this assessment procedure. At the end of the 10-minute period, the parent would announce that an assessment had occurred and would state the number of stutters that were noted. John earned two dollars for each assessment period that contained less than 0.5 %SS.[1]

Because John had not shown complete generalization after the conclusion of the ELU program, a sequential modification program was devised (see Table 1, page 54). A hierarchy of six speaking situations was selected, and John was given the task of obtaining four 2,000-syllable tape recordings containing less than 0.5 %SS in each of those situations. The

---

[1] John's parents were familiar with his speech rate, so it was possible to estimate the number of stutterings to occur in a 10-minute period which would exceed the 0.5 %SS criterion.

situations chosen for the hierarchy were as follows, in order from least to most difficult: Talking to his sister; talking to the local shopkeeper; talking to a specified teacher in private; talking to a stranger; talking in front of his scout group; making telephone enquiries. Each tape recording was presented for assessment to his parents. If the recording of him in that speaking situation was below 0.5 %SS, and contained 2,000 syllables, then John was permitted to attempt another recording in that situation. Above 0.5 %SS on a tape meant that John was to return to the first recording in that situation.[1] When John had successfully completed four consecutive, stutter-free recordings in a situation, then he was permitted to attempt the next situation. John's parents offered a substantial reward for his completion of this generalization program.

In addition to its possible value in promoting generalization, the sequential modification program was designed to facilitate a shift in management responsibility toward the family. While this sequential modification program was being completed, John and his father attended the clinic only once per week to report on progress and to receive guidance from the clinician (they attended twice per week during the Instatement Phase). However, phone contact was maintained at specified times during the week. This procedure was consistent with the stated management plan for John's treatment, where responsibility for management would shift to his parents. This portion of management required much encouragement from the clinician to ensure that the family persevered with the tasks. On one occasion John and both parents were scheduled for a clinic visit, specifically for the purpose of counselling, after 3 weeks had elapsed without completion of any assignments.

John succeeded with his sequential modification program after 11 weeks. He found the phone enquiry assignment particularly difficult, and experienced many failed recordings. However, the clinician was confident that John had sufficient speech skills to succeed in the task, and—providing he received the support of his parents—allowed him to encounter these failures in the interests of improving his speech skills. Some weeks before John had completed the program, beyond- and within-clinic recordings showed that his stuttering rate was consistently at or below 10 stutters per 2,000 syllables (0.5 %SS). Several surprise telephone calls by the clinician confirmed this result. John was then admitted to a maintenance program because he had met the criterion that was established during the Instatement Phase.

### The Maintenance Phase of treatment

Johns' maintenance target was less than or equal to 10 stutters in 2,000-syllable conversations. This criterion was applied to within- and beyond-clinic tapes. The clinician considered that no criteria other than this were necessary for John.

A performance-contingent maintenance program (see page 62, Table 2) was devised with 10 steps. At each step, John was required to complete two 2,000-syllable clinic tasks; conversation with a clinician and conversation on the telephone. For the week preceding each maintenance visit, John was required to complete two 2,000-syllable beyond-clinic recordings of conversations; one with his brother, and another with a non-family member at each maintenance visit. In order to pass a maintenance step, all these recordings and clinic conversations were required to contain 2,000 syllables with 10 or fewer stutters. John's parents were required to assess his beyond-clinic tapes, although the clinician checked these carefully.

---

[1] If a recording did not contain sufficient syllables, this did not mean a return to the first recording. Instead, John was required to re-attempt that recording.

After the maintenance program was under way, the clinician decided that it would be best if the family actually visited the clinic only at a few steps; at M3, M8, and M10. For the remainder of the maintenance steps, the family did not come to the clinic. The two 2,000-syllable tapes were mailed to the clinician for checking. In place of within-clinic conversations, the clinician telephoned John and rated his speech on-line. The same stuttering rate performance criterion applied for these phone conversations. With these "distance" arrangements, John was told that if he did not succeed in any maintenance step he would visit the clinic for the resulting M1 assessment.

John completed this program with two failed maintenance assessments. With the latter of these, John was discouraged by having to return to the start of the program. However, the clinician discussed with John and his parents the importance of adhering to a maintenance program and not waiving the performance criteria. In particular, it was pointed out that such a program was as much a part of John's treatment as any preceding phase. In fact, the clinician stated that such a program, properly administered, probably was the single most important component of adequate stuttering treatment.

*Follow-up*

One year after John completed the maintenance program, his case was followed up by the clinician. This was a routine procedure for all clients, to assess the long-term benefits of the stuttering treatments provided by the clinic. At a clinic visit, the family stated that there had been several slight relapse problems during the year. However, the clinician was pleased to hear that the family had felt well equipped to handle those problems without needing to consult the clinic.

John was able to conduct two conversations with the clinician with less than his target of 0.5 %SS, and two beyond-clinic tape recordings from the previous week showed equally good speech performance. John's family assisted him to complete a questionnaire about his perception of how useful his treatment had been. Some of John's responses on this questionnaire indicated that he thought the program "very much" worthwhile. Further, he responded that he was "very satisfied" with his speech after treatment and at the time of follow-up. John indicated that he currently attends to the task of producing stutter-free speech in "fewer than 1/10 of daily speech situations." Further, John indicated that he had improved in self confidence since the treatment program.

# Example Two:
# Programmed prolonged-speech treatment

## Background

A clinician who specialized in stuttering treatments received a referral of Jeff, a 15-year-old boy, who presented with a one-year history of unsuccessful treatment with an ELU program. Repeatedly, Jeff succeeded in instating stutter-free speech, and then achieved only partial success in systematic generalization tasks. Jeff's parents felt that the lack of success in generalization caused him to lose motivation to continue with the treatment. He had never been instructed in the use of prolonged speech to eliminate stuttered speech. The ELU program was the only treatment that he had received, and his previous clinician had not incorporated prolonged speech into that treatment as recommended by Costello (1983).

In the clinic, Jeff's stuttering was severe. The clinician recorded 23.5 %SS and 120 SPM during a 1,000-syllable conversation. Long blocks and prolongations occurred, accompanied by grimacing and facial twitching. Jeff reported that speaking was effortful, and described feelings of constriction in the throat when attempting to speak. Jeff and his parents said that he was apprehensive about certain speaking situations, and often experienced a long block when attempting to speak in those situations. Those troublesome situations included telephone conversations with strangers, answering questions in class, and shopping. Jeff's parents believed that his stuttering had gradually worsened over the past three years.

### The Preliminary Phase

The clinician decided that a treatment based on prolonged speech would be suitable. This decision was made for several reasons. First, the clinician was satisfied that the ELU program was ineffective in controlling Jeff's stuttering without the addition of any features of prolonged speech. Second, it was considered that, alone, operant procedures would be of limited use, because little of Jeff's speech was free of stuttering. Finally, the clinician thought it possible that Jeff might have a severe and chronic stuttering problem if a successful means of control was not established promptly.

The clinician told Jeff's parents that prolonged speech treatment would be advisable, and also pointed out that this treatment is not always successful with 15-year-olds. The clinician described intensive prolonged speech treatment, and suggested this as a possible future option.

### The Instatement Phase of treatment

Jeff's treatment combined prolonged speech with the ELU procedure. The clinician demonstrated the skills of "gentle onsets" and "soft contacts" (see page 100), which Jeff acquired readily. Then, Jeff worked through the stages of the ELU program using those skills to succeed at treatment tasks. The clinician's intention was for him to achieve 5 minutes of stutter-free speech, and then to assess speech quality and shape natural sounding speech if necessary. However, the clinician found that, at the 2-minute level of the program, Jeff's prolonged speech had become natural sounding. Hence, treatment tasks contained no specific goal of natural sounding prolonged speech.

Jeff progressed consistently through the ELU program steps, which were conducted by his parents in two half-hour sessions each day. The clinician regularly viewed video tape recordings of these home sessions, and was satisfied that they were conducted properly by the parents. In five weeks Jeff achieved the ELU treatment goal of five minutes of stutter-free conversation. His speech at that time during treatment trials was scored as "3" on the speech naturalness scale, which sounded quite natural to the clinician and Jeff's parents. Further, Jeff stated that he felt comfortable using prolonged speech in treatment trials with his parents. In consultation, Jeff, his parents, and the clinician determined that a zero stuttering criterion would be attempted for the remainder of the treatment.

Stutter-free speech showed signs of generalizing partially to situations other than treatment trials. Each day, Jeff's father used a 10-point severity scale (see Part Two) to covertly assess his speech for a randomly chosen 5-minute interval. These severity scores showed a decrease from an average rating of 8.2 in the first week of treatment to an average rating of 2.3 in the fourth week of treatment. Additionally, the clinician conversed with Jeff for 1,000 syllables at the start of each clinic visit. At the third clinic visit, Jeff used prolonged speech during this conversation without being asked to do so, and stuttered only once or twice. Jeff's parents reported that, since the beginning of prolonged speech instruction, he had not experienced any severe blocks in speaking situations which he usually found troublesome. In those situations, Jeff was using prolonged speech. The clinician believed that several factors contributed to Jeff's excellent progress. First, his parents were dedicated to the treatment program, and had become skilled in conducting treatment trials. They also generally encouraged him to use prolonged speech in everyday situations, and praised him when he did so. Jeff's parents also devised systematic tangible rewards for him as he progressing through different stages of the program. Finally, Jeff was particularly intelligent and motivated.

When Jeff had achieved five minutes of stutter-free conversational speech with his parents, clinic visits ceased for one month. During this month, Jeff was required to maintain his skill of producing five minutes of conversational, stutter-free speech. Three times each day he attempted a treatment trial, and his parents kept a record of the number of his successful treatment trials. The purpose of this record was to detect any gradual loss of Jeff's speech skills. The clinician's rationale for prescribing this one-month period was that there would be nothing to gain, but everything to lose, in proceeding rapidly through a treatment program. It was feared that Jeff might lose his enthusiasm for it. Additionally, the clinician reasoned that the generalization of stutter-free speech that had occurred to date might continue without formal generalization procedures. Throughout this month, the parents made telephone contact with the clinician each week.

During the month Jeff did not lose his prolonged speech skills. In the first week he succeeded in producing zero stuttering in 19 of 21 trials, in the second week 17 out of 18 trials (three trials for one day were missed due to illness), and 20 out of 21 trials in the third and fourth weeks.

## The Generalization and Maintenance Phases

At the clinic appointment at the end of the month, the clinician discussed with Jeff's parents the following possible choices for continued management:

1. Extensive speech practice, perhaps in an intensive format.
2. A systematic generalization program based on sequential modification.
3. A program of surprise assessments linked to a reward system.
4. Continued monitoring of the effects of regular speech practice.

The clinician decided to design a generalization program based on sequential modification, and to follow that program with a performance contingent maintenance program. The rationale for this was that the parents' beyond-clinic SMST recordings, which they collected each week, showed the presence of significant levels of stuttering in everyday speech situations. Jeff had responded well to training of stutter-free speech with his parents, so it was considered possible that he would respond similarly to training of stutter-free speech in other situations. A sequential modification program similar to John's (see pages 109-110) was designed and implemented. At the conclusion of this program, beyond-clinic covert measures consistently showed stuttering rates at zero %SS. A maintenance program, also similar to John's was then designed and implemented.

# Part Five:

# Perspectives on Stuttering[1]

Ann Packman assisted with organizing the material in Part Five.

One reason why clinicians need to appreciate various perspectives on stuttering is that it can assist them to explain the condition to clients and parents. Explanations from different perspectives are necessary in different clinical situations. For example, some parents of stuttering children feel that they somehow are responsible for the disorder. In which case a clinician can draw on current views of the cause of stuttering to allay that misapprehension. Other parents may be apprehensive about drawing attention to stuttered speech, for fear that this will worsen the disorder. In which case the clinician can explain the known beneficial effects of operant methodology on early stuttering.

Clinicians also need to incorporate perspectives of stuttering into their explanation of how a recommended treatment is supposed to stop or reduce stuttering. All treatments, especially those for adults, impose considerably on the lives of clients and their families, and require considerable motivation in order to be completed successfully. It is unrealistic to expect clients or their families to muster such efforts without a credible explanation of why they are engaging in certain activities. For example, a clinician who advises a client to practice "Stage 40 prolonged speech" (see Part Four) for a half-hour each day would need to have a good theoretical explanation for why that might help to control stuttering. Similarly, a clinician can hardly expect a parent to conduct daily 10-minute operant treatment sessions at home, plus provide regular on-line feedback to a young child (see Part Three), without explaining how those activities are expected to eliminate stuttered speech. And if a clinician recommends for a client a program of systematic relaxation, then an explanation is needed for how that might contribute to alleviating stuttered speech.

Theoretical perspectives on stuttering have a place in the accountability of treatment services offered to stuttering clients. Certainly, evaluating treatment outcome is a part of that accountability (see page 35). However, a clinician's accountability for treatment choice extends further than simply showing that the treatment works. The clinician also needs to make justifiable choices about which treatment to attempt in the first place. As Siegel and Ingham (1987) argue, it is not sufficient to conduct clinical practice with a belief that any treatment that "works" is satisfactory. Clinicians cannot uncritically accept any idea about how to treat stuttering, because clients need to be protected from useless—and perhaps even harmful—interventions. Stuttering has attracted some extraordinary and not particularly credible ideas about its treatment, such as Summers' (1986) suggestion of "handwriting therapy." Another example is surgery of the tongue (see Van Riper, 1973). One way to establish that such treatment ideas are of little value is to reject them as unjustifiable from established perspectives on the disorder.

Another important reason for clinicians to have perspectives on stuttering is that they play a role in day-to-day clinical practice. Every treatment session contains an endorsement of some view of stuttering. For example, the treatment for early stuttering recommended in Part Three emphasizes an operant perspective of the disorder. Another example is where clinicians regard stuttering as a speech motor control problem and use a prolonged speech treatment to compensate for that problem. It is critical to be aware of the role of such theoretical perspectives in daily treatment practices, because those perspectives will eventually become less favored, and treatment practices will change accordingly. The following sections contain examples of perspectives on stuttering which are in various stages of changing favor and disfavor. Perhaps the best example considered in the following sections is the waning popularity of the diagnosogenic theory. That change has dramatically affected the way clinicians treat young stuttering children. Several such changes are likely to occur during the course of any clinician's career.

In what follows, some perspectives are given only a cursory overview because the period of their influence has past. However, other perspectives, such as operant methodology, anxiety, genetics, and the environment, are treated in more detail because they are particularly relevant to clinical practices.

# Operant Methodology

One perspective on stuttering is its control with operant methodology. Explorations of stuttering and operant methodology have traditionally been completely atheoretical, being merely descriptions of the various ways that environmental events can control stuttered speech. In fact, the experimental analysis of behavior as developed by Skinner disavows even theoretical constructs such as "anxiety," "drive," and "avoidance" which feature in other perspectives on stuttering:

> The experimental analysis of behavior involves the systematic manipulation of stimulus and response conditions in order to identify unambiguous functional relationships between behavior and environmental events. The procedures used to establish this relationship require the identification of a response class, the use of frequency or response rate as the experimental datum, and the investigation of the individual organism (Ingham, 1984, p. 200)

This highlights the important point that stuttering is not an "operant." To be an operant, a behavior needs to be created and maintained by environmental consequences. As Ingham (1984) points out, there is no such implication behind the experimental analysis of stuttering behavior.[1]

It is not the purpose of this section to review the considerable body of literature dealing with the effects of response contingent stimulation (RCS) on stuttering. Such reviews can be found in a number of places (Bloodstein, 1987; Costello & Ingham, 1984b; Nittrouer & Cheney, 1984; Prins & Hubbard, 1988). Instead, this section overviews some landmark studies in operant methodology and stuttering, and some studies which have particular relevance to clinical practice.

## The seminal study

A set of within-subject experiments by Flanagan, Goldiamond, and Azrin (1958) is generally recognized as the first demonstration of the operant properties of stuttering. Three adult subjects received RCS for 30 minutes subsequent to displaying a stable baseline. This was followed by a further 30-minute baseline phase. Subjects were studied with this ABA design on two consecutive days. On one day a 1-second, 105 dB tone was presented contingent on each stuttering. On another of the days negative reinforcement was used; the tone was continuous but removed for 5 seconds contingent on each stuttering. Results showed that stuttering rates increased or decreased with the application of RCS, and returned to baseline levels when RCS was withdrawn. Subsequent to the Flanagan, Goldiamond, and Azrin (1958) study, Martin and colleagues were involved in many RCS experiments at the University of Minnesota which incorporated various stimuli with adult subjects (for example, Martin & Berndt, 1970; Martin & Haroldson, 1971; 1977; Martin & Siegel, 1966a; 1966b; Martin, St. Louis, Haroldson, & Hasbrouck, 1975).

---

[1] There is much confusion on this point in the field (see Ingham, 1984; Prins & Hubbard, 1988). According to Ingham (1975), much of that confusion can be traced to two attempts to explain stuttering as an operant; Shames and Sherrick (1963) and Goldiamond (1965).

# Operant methodology with early stuttering

One of the most notable studies in stuttering research occurred when Martin, Kuhl and Haroldson (1972) experimentally applied RCS to the stuttering of two preschool-age children. The success of this experiment was a landmark in providing a new way to think about early stuttering and how it might be managed clinically. The experiment used a time-out (TO) stimulus applied with the ingenious device of a talking puppet which was mounted and illuminated in a box. Hence, this study sometimes is referred to as the "puppet study." Each child sat in a room and conversed with the puppet, which was operated from outside the room by an experimenter. Following a baseline consisting of a number of 20-minute conversations with this puppet, it "disappeared" contingent on stuttering. With one of the children, TO initially was presented contingent on stuttering longer than 2 seconds. In a later phase, TO was presented contingent on each stutter. For both children, immediate stuttering reductions occurred during the TO condition, and generalized to "probe sessions" in the laboratory, where the children conversed with an adult. Some follow-up data suggested that these gains were maintained after one year.

From a clinical perspective, the study is of interest because of its challenge to the diagnosogenic theory. It suggested that direct stimulation would facilitate recovery from stuttering in young children, not worsen the condition. Further, it demonstrated that RCS can be presented in a format that is both ethical and practicable for use with young children. As provocative as the results of the puppet study might be, they should be considered with serious reservations because the experiment did not show convincingly that the stuttering of the children was controlled by the TO procedure. Another concern about the study is that its results have not been replicated or expanded. One possible exception is a study by Reed and Godden (1977) with two children, aged 3 years and 5 years. The stimulus "slow down" was presented contingent on stuttering and appeared to eliminate stuttering. However, these results are compromised by the nature of the stimulus; it is not clear whether "slow down", in fact, prompted the subjects to eliminate stuttering by reducing speech rate. Also, Reed and Godden used a multiple baseline across subjects design, but the use of only two subjects weakened the findings. This issue of absence of replication of the puppet study is resumed in a later section which deals with the choice of a treatment for early stuttering.

# Self-managed response contingent stimulation

Some of the most clinically important studies of the operant nature of stuttering have concerned the self-administration of contingencies for stuttered speech. Such procedures are easy for clients to learn, and to apply in their everyday speaking environments. There is every reason to believe that such techniques would make a useful contribution to "mediating generalization" of treatment effects (see Part Two).

After a single 30-minute conversational baseline session, La Croix (1972) instructed two subjects to use a hand-held counter to record the number of stutters during subsequent sessions (20 sessions for one subject and 14 for the other). Both subjects reduced stuttering rates to near zero. Although this finding is particularly provocative, it is weakened by the omission of speech rate data. Further, the frequency of the experimental sessions was not reported. No direct replication of the study has been reported to date.

Martin and Haroldson (1982) reported a study where subjects spoke in six 10-minute speaking sessions which involved telephone, monologue, and monologue with TO. Thirty subjects spoke under each of these conditions. However, 10 subjects received experimenter-administered TO (EATO), 10 subjects received subject-administered TO (SATO), and 10 control subjects received no TO. Findings showed that SATO and EATO produced equivalent reductions in stuttering. In other words, the effects of time-out were not dependent on a clinician. However, after a second TO period it was clear that SATO generalized its effects into a subsequent telephone conversation, but EATO did not. This result verified that—as might be expected—self-managed time-out may facilitate generalization of treatment effects.

Another interesting finding in the Martin and Haroldson study was the relation between the effects of SATO and the subjects' self-monitoring accuracy. For SATO conditions, average point-to-point agreement between subjects and experimenters on stutters was only 76.6 percent. Further, data from individual subjects showed no systematic relationship between self-monitoring accuracy and the effect of TO. In other words, the effects of self-administered TO were not dependent on experimenter-subject agreement in stuttering identification.

The relation between self-monitoring accuracy and the effects of self monitoring was explored also by James (1981a). Thirty-three stuttering subjects were divided into groups according to accuracy on a self monitoring task; high accuracy (74 percent), medium accuracy (51 percent), and low accuracy (26 percent). The findings in the Martin and Haroldson (1982) study were replicated. In fact, self monitoring accuracy was *negatively* correlated with the amount of stuttering reduction obtained by self monitoring; the subjects who were least accurate in self monitoring benefited most from the procedure. One important feature of this study was that a small number of subjects (4) were able to eliminate more than 70 percent of their stuttering with self monitoring. Eight subjects increased stuttering in response to the procedure.

James (1981b) demonstrated the potential clinical value of the self-imposed TO procedure with a single subject using a multiple baseline across situations design. In the first part of the study, a subject who stuttered learned to self-impose TO contingent on stuttering. Then this procedure was applied in a variety of usual speaking situations, with the result that clinically significant stuttering reductions occurred in those situations. In the second part of the study, a similar multiple baseline design across situations was used, but the response studied was accuracy of self-initiated TO. Within and beyond the clinic, a response-cost procedure was used to punish failure to self-impose TO. Results showed that reliability of the subject's self-initiation of TO increased from 45.5 percent to 62.8 percent agreement with the examiner. A striking effect of this improved self monitoring skill was that stuttering within and beyond the clinic decreased to near zero. Further, these stuttering reductions remained when the response cost procedure was withdrawn. Data showed that these stuttering reductions occurred without compromising speech rate. At 6 and 12 months follow-up, the subject had maintained these near-zero stuttering rates.

The few studies reviewed above give the impression that researchers prefer punishment of stuttered speech to reinforcement of stutter-free speech. This seems to be because punishment is more effective than reinforcement in controlling stuttering.[1] Further, reviewers of the operant literature on stuttering have noted that the TO stimulus seems to be the one with the most powerful controlling effects on the disorder. In light of this, some investigations by James, concerning the nature of the TO stimulus, are of considerable interest. James (1976) assigned 45 stuttering subjects to five groups, each of which experienced a different TO period duration during monologue; 1 second, 5 seconds, 10 seconds, and 30 seconds. The fifth group was a control. Surprisingly, findings indicated that

---

[1] However, in the case of operant methodology with children, punishment has serious limitations, as considered in Part Three.

the duration of the TO stimulus was irrelevant to the effect of the procedure. In another study concerning the nature of TO, James (1981c) placed 36 stuttering subjects into four groups; contingent TO, non-contingent TO (TO was presented randomly), contingent tone (a tone was presented contingent on stuttering), and non-contingent tone (the tone was presented randomly). Results indicated that the only effective stimulus for eliminating stuttering was the contingent TO. In other words, both the contingency of the stimulation and the TO stimulation were critical to the success of the procedure; presentation of a tone either contingently or noncontingently was not effective in reducing stuttering.[1] Another study (James, 1983) compared the effects of 10 seconds of experimenter-imposed TO, 10 seconds of self-imposed TO, and an experimenter-imposed TO condition where subjects could terminate the TO interval when they wished. All conditions produced identical reductions of stuttering rate in 33 subjects (around 50 percent of baseline stuttering rates). However, this study was consistent with the James (1981a) study in that a number of subjects were found who eliminated the majority of stuttering with the TO procedure; 5 subjects reduced stuttering by more than 80 percent. A particularly interesting feature of this study was that subjects who could choose the duration of their TO interval chose an average of less than two seconds, which is quite a manageable interval for self-imposed TO during everyday conversations.

## Stuttering and operant methodology: Conclusions

There is no doubt from many laboratory studies that RCS can modify stuttering. Responses in those studies have included stuttering and stutter-free speech segments, and the controlling effects of a number of stimuli have been established. These findings are of enormous interest to clinicians, because they demonstrate a way to control stuttering without speaking with an unusual speech pattern. Further, their simplicity makes them suitable for stuttering control in children and easy for parents to learn. Three studies suggest that verbal RCS might be particularly useful in the control of early stuttering. Studies also demonstrate that self-managed RCS might be useful in the control of stuttering in some subjects, although the procedure does not produce clinically significant stuttering reductions for all subjects. Self-imposed TO seems to be a particularly powerful version of self managed RCS, which allows for some clinical flexibility because its benefits seem only to depend on the stimulation being contingent, not on the accuracy of self monitoring or the duration of the TO period. These findings suggest that direct application of RCS, self-managed RCS, and operant shaping are important clinical techniques.

## Operant treatment research

It is peculiar that research findings showing the value of operant treatments for stuttering have been generally overlooked, despite their considerable clinical implications. This may be because of the methodology used in that research. The within-subject methodology in this line of enquiry has been eschewed by some influential reviewers of stuttering treatment literature. For example, Bloodstein's (1987) criteria for assessing treatment effectiveness specifies that only group research designs, not single-subject designs, are admissible sources of evidence. And in effect, Andrews, Guitar, and Howie's (1980) well known assessment of treatment effectiveness overlooked single-subject reports. The reason

---

[1] Ingham (1984) has argued that there is a methodological problem with this study which weakens the finding that the contingent tone did not produce stuttering reductions.

for this is that Andrews et al. used a meta-analysis, which is a statistical procedure designed to compare the sizes of treatment effects associated with different procedures. Unfortunately, though, the meta-analysis can only include data from group-based clinical trial designs, so this influential report inadvertently de-emphasized pertinent within-subject research.

Another reason why the clinical relevance of within-subject research may have been overlooked is that it does not focus on treatment outcome. That is not the main power of that research design. Instead, the power of such studies is that they are able to establish clinically relevant variables which may be used to control stuttering. For example, some studies previously overviewed which have shown the controlling effects of time-out and self-monitoring. It is arguable that these findings make more of a contribution to clinical practice than group studies of the effectiveness of treatments, because they provide information about variables which can control stuttering and which clinicians can use creatively in designing treatments. At present, research has established a great deal about the treatment process with operant treatments, but relatively little about the outcome of those treatments. Posttreatment periods of around one year are probably the minimum requisite for adequate outcome evaluation, but there have been few studies with methodological credentials to assess any such long-term effects of treatment.

A number of studies have investigated the effects of treatments which are specifically built around RCS. It is beyond the scope of this text to review these studies individually, but they are organized for reference in Table 3 according to the age of the subjects, and the kind of RCS which they used. The table includes only studies for which speech data were presented in support of claims of treatment effects. Some laboratory studies of RCS and stuttering have been included in Table 3 if they either show evidence of generalization of treatment effects to outside the laboratory or demonstrate near-zero stuttering levels achieved for many experimental sessions with clinical rather than laboratory apparatus. Laboratory studies involving noxious stimuli such as shock or loud noise are not included.

An overlooked fact about advanced stuttering is that, for some clients, it might be controllable with simple, nonprogrammed treatments. James' (1981a, 1983) studies concerning self-adminstered RCS suggest that around 10 percent of adults may benefit from these procedures. That information is bolstered by a number of other findings, such as La Croix's (1973) demonstration of the potential power of self-counts of stuttering, and James' (1981b) report of the clinical application of self-imposed TO. Taken together, these findings leave little doubt that a number of adult clients will benefit from management based on nonprogrammed RCS. This is not to say that the number of such clients is large. It might be a small portion of cases of advanced stuttering who benefit from such procedures. But the point is that such clients exist and must be identified so that they can receive an operant treatment as a first management strategy rather than a prolonged-speech treatment. As mentioned before, there are many advantages to simple treatments; they facilitate self-management, they do not result in speech which sounds unnatural, and they do not take as long to complete. It would be an error to treat a client with prolonged speech if that client's stuttering could be controlled with a simpler procedure.

TABLE THREE. Treatment reports involving response contingent stimulation. Preschool = below 5 years, child = 6-12 years, adolescent = 13-16 years,
adult = greater than 16 years. RC = response cost (contingent removal of
token) SH = shaping (GILCU or a variant such as ELU), CO = counting of
stutters, SI = self-imposed RCS, TO = time out, TR = tangible reward, VP =
verbal punishment, VR = verbal reward.

| Study | Age | Procedure/s |
|-------|-----|-------------|
| Martin, Kuhl, & Haroldson (1972) | preschool | TO |
| Onslow, Andrews, & Lincoln (in press) | preschool | TR, VP, VR |
| Onslow, Costa, & Rue (1990) | preschool, child | TR, VP, VR |
| Reed & Godden (1977) | preschool, child | VP |
| Rickard & Mundy (1965) | child | SH, TR |
| Leach (1969) | child | TR |
| Shaw & Shrum (1972) | child | TR, |
| Manning, Trutna, & Shaw (1976) | child | TR, VP |
| Salend & Andress (1984) | child | RC |
| Johnson, Coleman & Rasmussen, (1978) | child | SH |
| Peters (1977) | child | TR |
| Martin & Berndt (1970) | child | TO |
| McDermott (1971) | child | SI, TO |
| Browning (1967) | child | VP, VR |
| Ryan (1970, 1971, 1974, 1981), Ryan & Van Kirk Ryan (1983) | child, adult | RC, SH, SI, TA, TR, VP, VR , TO |
| Mowrer (1975) | child, adult | SH |
| Costello (1984) | child | SH, TO, VR |
| Costello (1975) | adolescent, adult | SI, TO, VR |
| James (1981b) | adult | SI, TO, CO |
| La Croix (1973) | adult | SI, CO |
| Ingham & Packman (1977) | adult | TO |
| James (1983) | adult | TO, SI |

# Speech
# Motor Control[1]

McClean (1990) refers to motor control as "how various centers and pathways of the brain contribute to the regulation of muscle contraction during natural behaviors" (p. 64). Netsell (1986) defines speech motor control as the "neuronal actions that initiate and regulate muscle contractions for speech production" (p. 89).

Starkweather (1987) has pointed out that a lot of what is known about stuttering can be explained in terms of speech motor control. He points out, for example, that stuttering occurs more frequently on stressed syllables, infrequent words, and at the beginning of sentences. Although those and other effects may reflect the role of linguistics in stuttering, it is just as easy to argue that demands on speech motor control are greater at such moments during speech. Starkweather also argues that various conditions that reduce stuttering (see Part One) might do so because they place less demands on speech motor control. Further, different stuttering rates in different speaking situations might reflect the different motor speech control requirements of those situations. The well known effects of fear and apprehension on stuttering could reflect the negative effects of such emotional variables on the complexities of speech motor control. As Starkweather indicates, subtle cognitive variables such as "self confidence" are known to influence the fine-tuning of performance in games such as tennis which require motor coordination.

A fundamental reason why stuttering can be considered as a speech motor control problem is because the condition involves motor dysfunction: There is obviously something wrong with speech-related movement. Perhaps that is why the earliest theories about the nature and cause of the condition focussed on speech motor function. Those theories are considered below.

## Early theories

Shortly after Lee Edward Travis formed the first academic speech-language pathology department at the University of Iowa (see Part Two), he and Samuel Orton presented the so-called Orton-Travis theory (Orton, 1927; Travis, 1931), otherwise known as the cerebral dominance theory. This is a well-known theory of the cause of stuttering, and its central premise is that the distal cause of stuttering is unestablished cerebral dominance for speech. Bryngelson, who was one of Travis' students, contributed to the development of the theory and was responsible for the development of "sidedness training" treatment. This technique involved the wearing of casts and slings on limbs, and various activities designed to correct the dominance problem of the disorder. Eventually this theory, and its associated treatments, were rejected in the face of mounting evidence that people who stutter are not atypical in their laterality.

Several other speech motor control theories were presented in the earlier decades of this century, but did not achieve any lasting influence. One of these was West's (1958) idea that

---

[1] This section was written with the assistance of Ann Packman.

stuttering is a convulsive disorder related to epilepsy, and mediated by blood sugar levels. Eisenson's (1958) perseverative theory was based on observations that linguistic and motor perseveration may occur following neurological insult. Perseveration is defined as "a tendency for a mental or motor act to persist, either in overt expression or in drive, for a longer than normal time after the stimulus that evoked the behavior has ceased to be present" (Eisenson, 1975, p. 403). Eisenson suggested that people who stutter have an abnormal tendency to do this, and that stuttered speech is caused by motor and linguistic perseveration.

# Cybernetic theories

Self-regulating machines do so with automatic control mechanisms called servosystems. Bloodstein (1987) outlines the various components of servosystems; a "sensor," feedback of information from the sensor, a controller unit with a "comparator" which compares intended output with actual output, and an "effector" which makes adjustments to output. Examples of servosystems are air-conditioning units and refrigerators. Cybernetics is the application of automatic control principles to engineering, biology and the social sciences. Examples of biological systems with servosystems are homeostatic mechanisms for body temperature and blood pressure.

The first of many cybernetic models of speech was proposed by Fairbanks (1954). At that time, feedback was thought to be critical in speech production. It was not surprising, then, that the discovery of the effects of delayed auditory feedback (DAF; see Part One) prompted the formulation of a set of cybernetic theories about the cause of stuttering (see Ingham, 1984). In 1950, Lee discovered that DAF disrupted normal speech (the "Lee effect"), and shortly after termed these speech disruptions "artificial stutter." However, it was subsequently clarified that DAF-induced speech disruptions are dissimilar to stuttered speech. A review of the subsequent research by Ingham (1984) indicates that the diverse effects of DAF include "nonfluency," reduced intelligibility, reduced speech rate, increased intensity, and increased phonation time. These effects depend largely on delay levels (usually between 50 to 250 msec), signal intensity levels, speaking rates and partially on age and sex of the speaker.

Fairbanks' cybernetic model of speech, combined with Lee's discovery and the DAF research it prompted, paved the way for a set of theories that incorporate the idea that stuttering is caused by defective feedback of the speech signal (for example, Mysak, 1960; Webster & Lubker, 1968). Such a line of reasoning was bolstered considerably by findings that masking noise, which removes air-conducted speech feedback, generally reduces stuttering (see Part One). Ingham (1984) has drawn attention to several problems with cybernetic theories of stuttering. First, the relevance of the effects of DAF to speech production models is questionable; the disruptive effects of DAF do not necessarily mean that nondisrupted speech depends on intact feedback. Second, the variable effects of DAF make it difficult to accept that there is a direct link between auditory feedback and speech production. Finally, it is common for stuttering blocks to occur on initial sounds of utterances, before any speech has occurred that could be disrupted.[1]

After a period of extensive research into masking and DAF, there have been comparatively few recent experimental reports concerning a servosystem view of stuttering. Certainly, a generally accepted theory has not emerged from research in this area. Perhaps

---

[1] See Perkins (1983b) for an ingenious way of getting around this objection.

this has been because of the many objections that can be raised against defective-servosystem theories. Recently, Postma and Kolk (1992) attempted to find experimental evidence that stuttering is a disorder of defective speech feedback. Those authors explained that the postulated problem in cybernetic theories is that the defective feedback results in the perception that a speech error has occurred when in fact no error has occurred. Stuttered speech is the speaker's attempt to correct the falsely perceived error. Postman and Kolk argued that this would mean that those who stutter would be less accurate than controls when monitoring their own phonetic errors, and that they would become more accurate when attempting to monitor errors in the presence of masking noise. Control and stuttering subjects read difficult phonetic sequences and monitored their production errors on-line. No performance differences were found between experimental and control subjects to support the experimental hypothesis. Further, stuttering subjects did not improve their error monitoring accuracy in the presence of masking noise.

# Models of stuttering

Research supports the notion that stuttering is a problem with speech motor control. Findings about people who stutter in relation to people who do not stutter are summarized as follows (these areas are covered in reviews by Adams, 1985; Bloodstein, 1987; Moore, 1984; 1990; Onslow & Ingham, 1987; Starkweather, 1982, 1987):

1. They have more involvement of the non-dominant cerebral hemisphere during processing of verbal material.
2. They have slower voice reaction times.
3. They have atypical aerodynamic, laryngeal, articulatory, EMG and acoustic activity during stutter-free speech.
4. They respond differently to certain non-speech tasks, such as tests of central auditory functioning, neuropsychological abilities, and overall motor abilities.

It is beyond the scope of this book to review all these findings, but they implicate speech motor control in stuttering. Not surprisingly, this research has prompted many theoretical explanations of how speech motor processes are involved in stuttering.

One way of theorizing about a system is to present a model of its inner workings by inference from what is known about its output. The value of such models is that they are useful for theorizing about causal factors which are unknown, and they are useful when the inner workings of a system cannot be measured directly. The latter two conditions pertain to the disorder of stuttering, so it is this type of model which has been used to try to explain stuttering in terms of speech motor control.

Martin Schwartz developed an *aerodynamic model* of stuttering which proposed that the stuttering block is essentially a laryngeal event (Schwartz, 1974; 1976). Schwartz suggested that stuttering is triggered by high subglottic pressure and that people who stutter have difficulty inhibiting the action of the posterior cricoarytenoid muscle (PCA) during speech. The action of the PCA is to abduct the vocal folds. Thus the model suggests that stuttering is caused by conflict between speech, which requires the vocal folds to adduct, and the action of the PCA, which causes the vocal folds to abduct. According to Schwartz's model, once this blockage has occurred the speaker may adopt compensatory or struggle behavior either at the laryngeal level, or above.

Schwartz used his model to make the prediction that stuttering would not occur at the top of the Empire State Building because of the drop in atmospheric pressure. He claimed that this prediction held true for one of his clients although he produced no data to support this claim (Scwartz, 1976). Schwartz claimed also that the model was verified with a treatment procedure called "flow and slow." It was claimed that by using this procedure the speaker can decrease subglottic pressure by starting airflow before commencing a phrase and then saying the first syllable of the phrase in a prolonged fashion.[1] However, Schwartz's (1976) claim that this treatment was successful was not substantiated empirically.

Neilson and colleagues (Andrews, Feyer, Hoddinott, Howie, & Neilson, 1983; Neilson & Neilson, 1987) have proposed an *adaptive sensory-motor processing model*. It explains stuttering as a central nervous system deficit which results in a "diminished ability to deal with the relationship between motor activity and the associated sensory or afferent activity produced during speech" (Andrews et al, 1983; p. 239). The model suggests that the output of speech motor activity is stored centrally to allow for comparison with the feedback signal. Neilson (1987) suggested that people who stutter have difficulty forming such an internal auditory-kinesthetic template against which the speech output is compared, and are obliged instead to produce speech using extra "central capacity" (Andrews et al, 1983, p. 239). Stuttering is said to occur because the speaker is obliged to spend more time comparing the feedback with the actual production.

In addition to findings that people who stutter have unusual right hemisphere activity during speech, there have been reports that such activity correlates with severity and is reduced by treatment (Boberg, Yeudall, Schopflocher, & Bo-Lassen, 1983; Moore, 1986). These data led Moore and Haynes (1980) to offer a "segmentation dysfunction hypothesis," where the left hemisphere is thought to be defective in fulfilling its normal role in the processing of speech and language. An elaboration of this idea is Yeudall's (1985) *neuropsychological model* of stuttering, which suggests that the non-dominant cerebral hemisphere of people who stutter gains executive control prior to or during speech production. Yeudall suggested that this may be due to insufficient activity in the dominant hemisphere or overactivity in the non-dominant hemisphere. Because people who stutter do not demonstrate any other signs of dominant hemisphere dysfunction, the second alternative is thought to be more likely. The cause could either be a structural lesion, or a functional disturbance such as a neurotransmitter imbalance. Yeudall emphasized the "gating" role of the thalamus during speech for both afferent and efferent signals. He hypothesized that when the nondominant hemisphere gains control of motor speech output, it switches the thalamic gate to redirect afferent signals. Yeudall suggested that stuttering is a result of this inappropriate gating and that struggle behavior, such as breath holding, may reflect inappropriate subcortical activity modulating brainstem centres rather than adaptive behavior.

Zimmerman and colleagues (Zimmerman, 1980; Zimmermann, Smith & Hanley, 1981) have developed a speech motor control model around the idea that people who stutter have normal speech mechanisms which are nonetheless prone to destabilization. The model suggests that stuttering is a result of excessive input to the motorneurone pools which regulate the reflex activity required for speech. This excessive input may come from environmental, emotional or physiological factors. It is suggested that this overloading of reflex activity may affect supralaryngeal, laryngeal and/or respiratory functions. Zimmerman (1980) predicted that certain postures of the articulators were a prerequisite for people who stutter to produce "fluent" utterances. These postures included decreased

---

[1] This treatment appears to be a variant of prolonged speech.

velocity and increased duration of articulatory movements. Zimmerman and Hanley (1983) investigated this notion using the fluency-enhancing condition of adaptation. They found that absence of stuttering was not necessarily accompanied by these postures. This finding led Zimmerman and Hanley to adjust the model to eliminate the causal relationship between the variables.

# Speech motor control and stuttering: Final comments

The extent of current interest in speech motor control and stuttering is reflected in the publication of two recent volumes devoted to the topic (Peters & Hulstijn, 1987; Peters, Hulstijn, & Starkweather, 1991). However, there is a caveat to the knowledge that certain speech motor anomalies are peculiar to stuttering. That caveat is that it implies nothing about the cause of stuttering. The features of a disorder are not necessarily related to its cause. In discussing the matter of unusual hemispheric processing in stuttering, Ingham (1989) has commented that observed anomalies could simply be a *result* of stuttering rather than its cause. The same comment pertains to voice reaction times, unusual EMG activity, and other more direct measures of speech motor function (Starkweather, 1990). Those anomalies may simply be the result of people struggling with whatever the fundamental aberration of stuttering might be. Research has yet to explore this matter.

# Genetics

## Basic terminology and concepts

"Proband" refers to a person affected with a disorder who is of immediate interest, or who presents to genetic investigators. "First degree relatives" are parents, siblings, or children of a proband. "Vertical transmission" is where an affected parent increases the risk of a child having a disorder. Evidence of vertical transmission is essential to any genetic explanation of transmission of a characteristic or disorder. "Monozygotic" (or identical) twins are genetically identical, and therefore always of the same sex. "Dizygotic" (fraternal, or nonidentical) twins have the same substantial genetic similarity as any other siblings, but happen to be conceived at the same time. "Concordance" refers to cases where both twins of a pair have a characteristic; stuttering in the present context. "Discordance" refers to cases where only one twin of the pair shows a characteristic. "Concordance rate" refers to the number of twin pairs that are concordant for a characteristic.

A "pedigree" is a coded graphical representation of a family which indicates the family members who display a characteristic or who are affected by a disorder. In a pedigree, the proband is indicated with an arrow. If a clinician constructs a pedigree of a client, it may be that the proband is the only family member that the clinician diagnoses as having the disorder. Other family members in the pedigree may be identified by the recall of the proband. An example of a pedigree of a client who stutters is presented in Figure 8, where first- and second-degree relatives are reported to be affected by the disorder. In that figure, squares represent males and circles represent females. Horizontal lines above family members represent sibling relationships, and horizontal lines below family members represent child-bearing relationships. Filled-in squares and circles indicate relatives that the client reports are currently stuttering or have ever been diagnosed as stuttering. Crosses indicate children younger than 5 years who reportedly are not stuttering. The client's partner's side of the pedigree in Figure 8 is not presented because no cases of stuttering were recalled.

FIGURE EIGHT: A hypothetical pedigree of a stuttering client with first- and second-degree relatives who are reported to be affected by stuttering. See text for explanation.

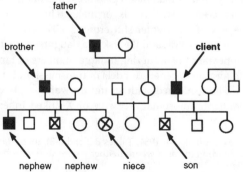

"Genotype" refers to a person's genetic constitution, and "phenotype" is the observable features of the person. Kidd (1984) notes that genetics plays a role in human development, but the relation between genotype and phenotype is complex, and nongenetic factors are undoubtedly involved in stuttering:

> The statement that heredity can affect behavior does not negate the importance of environmental factors; behavioral traits are obviously affected by learning and by an individual's psychosocial environment ...complex behavioral disorders, such as stuttering, are not determined by nature or by nurture, but by both. (Kidd, 1984; p. 149)

In one strict sense of the word "environment," genetic and environmental influences can be conceptualized as the total of all influences that could be responsible for the development of stuttering. That strict sense of "environment" includes "chemical composition, temperature, biologic events such as infections" (Kidd, 1977). As considered in a later section, writers sometimes allude to a role played by the "environment" in the development of stuttering, but are referring only to cultural or learned factors as the "environment."

# Types of genetic research

Direct procedures for examining genes are available (Martin & Kinnear, 1985), but these methods have provided no data pertaining to stuttering. Investigations to date of the genetic aspects of stuttering have used three kinds of methodology, which are considered in the sections below.

## Family studies: The Yale Study

A major family study, under the direction of Kenneth Kidd, began at Yale University in 1973 and spanned a decade. Its results have appeared in numerous publications, and seem to constitute the bulk of knowledge about stuttering in families. In total, 600 people who stutter and thousands of first degree relatives were studied. About half the probands were assessed by a speech clinician, and half were identified with self-report questionnaire. All probands had stuttered for a minimum of six months at some time of life.

Findings of high incidence of stuttering among relatives of probands (see Kidd, 1984) suggested the presence of an inherited susceptibility to contract the disorder. There are fewer females who stutter, but the Yale data showed that female probands had higher numbers of stuttering relatives than males (Kidd, 1984). This is consistent with the disorder having *sex-modified expression*. In other words, females are more resistant to an inherited susceptibility to stutter, seeming to require more inherited genetic material for them to acquire the disorder. Nonetheless, females seem to pass on a genetic susceptibility to stuttering. More susceptibility, in fact, than males pass on, if the following summary figures (from Kidd, 1977) are given credibility: Overall for males who stutter, the risk of a son stuttering is 22%, and the risk of a daughter stuttering is 9.0%. Overall for females who stutter, the risk of a son stuttering is 36%, and the risk of a daughter stuttering is 17%.[1]

Data that depict the appearance of stuttering in large numbers of families over several generations can be used to formulate genetic models of transmission. It was found that the Yale family data could not be explained with straightforward single-gene transmission models of autosomal dominant, autosomal recessive or X-linked inheritance (see Kidd,

---

[1] In a number of places (for example, Kidd, 1984; Tables 8-2 and 8-3), these data are broken down further in terms of risk to children in cases where neither parent of the proband stuttered or the father of the proband stuttered.

1984). Kidd (1984) outlines two possible explanations for the Yale family data. These are mathematically based genetic models referred to as "single major locus" and "polygenic." Polygenic transmission involves a number of genes contributing a small amount to the inherited tendency. The single major locus model explains how a single gene interacts with nongenetic factors to explain family data.

In addition to supporting a genetic model, the Yale family data have been used to investigate two cultural, or learning, hypotheses of the development of stuttering. The first of these is transmission by mimicry. It is common in speech clinics to find parents who suspect that their child has "copied" stuttering from a sibling or another child. If mimicry is involved in some way in the etiology of stuttering, then children who stutter should not be randomly distributed among the birthranks. Earlier children in a family would have fewer models of stuttering to copy than children born later, and hence would begin to stutter less often than children later in birthranks. Gladstein, Seider, and Kidd (1981) used the Yale data to obtain records of 303 sibships where all siblings were above 14 years. Mean birthrank for stuttering siblings did not differ from the expected mean birthrank in a random distribution of siblings. A statistical test was applied to assess the difference in frequency of stutterers pre- and post-proband (for sibships where neither parent stuttered). Results indicated that the number of pre- and post-proband stutterers did not differ. In general, there was no evidence of atypical sibship patterns, therefore no support for cultural transmission through mimicry.

The second cultural, or learning hypothesis, about stuttering was investigated by Cox, Seider, and Kidd (1984). Those investigators assessed aspects of the case histories and living environments of 14 families that contained at least five people who stuttered ("high density" families). The study utilized a control group of 10 families without a member who stuttered. Extensive case histories were obtained for family members in the following areas; prenatal, medical, developmental, social, and educational. None of the case histories distinguished stuttering, recovered stuttering, nonstuttering, or control family members.

Four self-report inventories were applied to the experimental and control families: The S24 scale of attitude to speech communication, which was completed by all adults and children above 12 yrs; the Taylor Manifest Anxiety Scale (TMAS), which was completed by all adults; the Parent Behavior Inventory (PBI), which all adults and older children completed separately for their mother and father; the Child Trait Checklist (CTC), which is a semantic differential procedure which parents used to describe their children. Predictably, the S24 scale of attitude to speech communication showed differences between those who stuttered, recovered stutterers, nonstuttering family members, and controls. Nonstuttering family members and controls did not differ in S24 scores. The TMAS and PBI (for both mothers and fathers) showed no significant differences between experimental and control families. Results for the CTC (with one extreme family removed) also showed no difference between experimental and control families. In general, no support was found for familial factors, such as speech-related anxiety or negative attitudes to speech, that might cause a predisposition to stuttering.

## Twin studies

One problem with family studies is that first-degree relatives, who share genetic material, usually also share environments for some part of their lives. Hence family studies do not directly assess the contribution of genetic material in the development of stuttering, because patterns of familial transmission might also be explained by nongenetic influences in family environments. However, twin studies are able to assess the contribution made by genetics in the development of a characteristic, although they do not allow formulation of genetic models. The logic underlying twin studies is that if a characteristic is concordant more often in monozygotic twins than in dizygotic twins, then a genetic component in a disorder is suggested. On several occasions this reasoning has been applied to genetic research into stuttering.

If studies of concordance rates in monozygotic and dizygotic twins are used to make any inferences about nongenetic sources of stuttering which are environmental, then they involve an important assumption. That assumption is that any such environmental influences have an equivalent effect on the two twin types. However, it is conceivable that monozygotic twins might "share" an environment to a greater extent than dizygotic twins. As stated by Morris-Yates, Andrews, Howie, and Henderson (1990), the identical nature of monozygotic twins might lead their families to treat them more similarly than dizygotic twins, and the similarities between them might prompt them to interact with their environments in similar ways. Therefore, it is conceivable that any nongenetic influences precipitating stuttering might affect both of a monozygotic twin pair more often than they affect both of a dizygotic twin pair.[1] A further limitation of twin genetic studies is that "biased ascertainment" may occur (Kidd, 1984); concordant twin pairs are more likely than discordant twin pairs to be identified by an experimenter. Kidd notes that one way of controlling for the effects of biased ascertainment in studies is the use of a twin register. However, this methodology has not been employed in any twin study dealing with stuttering. Kidd therefore concludes that the results of twin studies should be interpreted with some caution.

A study by Howie (1981) is recognized as the most methodologically sound of a number of studies that have been reported to date. In formulating this study, Howie noted that previous studies had found higher monozygotic concordance rates for stuttering. However, these research efforts were compromised by a number of methodological weaknesses that could have biased results in favor of a genetic hypothesis. Fundamentally, determination of stuttering and zygosity[2] was not made independently, and those determinations were made using questionable criteria. Further, Howie notes that, in existing studies, same- and different-sexed dizygotic twin pairs were considered together. It is known that sex influences the development of stuttering, therefore such a methodology fails to control for this variable. Howie also notes that no previous study incorporated an assessment of any bias in ascertainment of twin pairs. Finally, previous studies had not considered the effects of age on concordance rates; the effects of "spontaneous recovery" (see Part One) in young children should be taken into account.

In Howie's study, 30 same-sexed twin pairs with at least one who stuttered were obtained, with a mean age of 13.5 years. Seventeen pairs were obtained from clinics and 13 pairs were obtained by advertisement. Zygosity was diagnosed using four criteria. Stuttering was diagnosed by a speech pathologist from 500-word samples of monologue and conversation.

"Proband-wise concordance rate" estimates the risk of stuttering in the twin of a stutterer. "Pairwise concordance rate" is the percentage of pairs where both twins stutter. Pairs 12 years or older were considered fully concordant, and younger pairs were weighted according to the Andrews and Harris (1964; see page 20) recovery rate data. As with previous studies, concordance was found to be higher with monozygotic than dizygotic

---

[1] Morris-Yates, Andrews, Howie, and Henderson (1990) conducted a study to adress this issue, and reported that "similar treatment imposed upon MZ twins on the basis of their zygosity alone is... not a threat to the validity of the twin method" (p. 322)

[2] It is not self-evident whether same-sexed twins are monozygotic or dizygotic, and there is a protocol for making such a determination.

pairs: 10/16 monozygotic pairs were concordant, with a corrected pairwise concordance rate of .63; 3/13 dizygotic pairs were concordant, with a corrected pairwise concordance rate of .19. Proband-wise concordance rates were .77 risk to a monozygotic twin of a stutterer and .32 risk to a dizygotic twin.

In order to assess for biases of ascertainment in the study, Howie compared frequency of concordance in the volunteer group with the clinic group of twins. Concordance rates were lower in the volunteer group, so it was claimed that "the volunteer group was free of the most serious source of sampling bias in twin studies: over-reporting of concordant MZ pairs" (p. 320). However, this claim might be questioned because concordance rates in the volunteer group were compared with a clinic group, but a clinic group may itself overestimate population concordance rates. Andrews, Morris-Yates, Howie, and Martin (1991) conducted a survey designed to assess whether existing twin data for stuttering overestimated concordance rates through sampling bias. Those authors obtained survey responses from 3,810 non-volunteer twin pairs who were enrolled on a twin register, of whom 3.2% of males and 1.2% of females reported "ever stuttering." Monozygotic concordance rates for stuttering in those respondents were found to be similar to those reported for twin studies which involved volunteer subjects. To assess the validity of their results, Andrews et al. telephoned two-thirds of the twins who reported "ever stuttering." Eighty-four percent of those twins were either heard to stutter on the telephone or, if they had recovered from stuttering, reported at some time seeking professional help or having the disorder interfere significantly with their lives.

### Separation studies

Studies of monozygotic twins reared apart are useful in evaluating the contribution of genetics in the development of human characteristics. The only available separation data for stuttering comes from a compilation of information concerning 95 known pairs of monozygotic twins reared apart (Farber, 1981). Five of these twin pairs reportedly contained a stutterer, and reportedly no pair was concordant. When considered alongside high concordance rates of monozygotic twins reared together, this report is particularly provocative. The reason is that it is the only genetic study which addresses what the nongenetic influences in the development of stuttering might be. As Bloodstein (1987) argues, the study suggests that the cultural and learning factors of a child's environment are involved in the origin of the disorder; if they are removed then monozygotic concordance rates are lowered.

One consideration in establishing the value of the Farber (1981) report is that its findings do not necessarily contradict those of monozygotic concordance in stuttering children reared together. Around one-third of monozygotic twin pairs reported in twin studies have been discordant, so the discordance in Farber's study may have been due to chance. Additionally, Farber's report was part of a 50-year retrospective study, and the observations about the presence or absence of stuttering were second hand.

# Clinical implications

A statement about the clinical relevance of genetic research in stuttering needs to acknowledge the limitations of that research. The issue of identification of stuttering is important in genetic research about stuttering, because its basic datum is whether or not individuals stutter. However, there is no completely satisfactory definition of the disorder (see Part One, and this raises a question about how reliably probands were identified in the Yale family data about stuttering (Ingham, 1990c). As noted by Pauls (1990), most first degree relatives of probands were not evaluated by the investigators, but were determined to be stuttering or not by the report of the proband. Yet no information is available about the agreement of relatives' recall and the judgment of a clinician about whether subjects stuttered. The potential informativeness of such a comparison is highlighted by the Howie (1981) twin study, where clinicians diagnosed 42 speakers as stuttering, but the mothers of nine of those speakers stated that the subject did not currently stutter. And in the same study, clinicians identified 18 subjects as not stuttering from speech samples, but the mothers of five of those subjects asserted that the subject either had the disorder at the time of the study or at some previous time.

There are currently no serious challenges to the conclusion that genetics plays some part in the development of stuttering. Precise risk estimates are available (see Footnote page 130), but these may not be accurate because of the limitations of existing data described above. In any event, certain children are considerably more at risk than others. Arguably, that information, coupled with information about the potential benefits of early intervention (see Part Two), compels clinicians to monitor certain children for the onset of stuttering; children or siblings of a stuttering client who are in or younger than the age range in which stuttering might begin. In other words, clinicians have the responsibility of prompt identification of the onset of stuttering in at-risk children, and also for deciding that at-risk preschool children are free of the disorder. This task is not a straightforward one, and how clinicians might accomplish it is discussed in detail in Part Seven.

# Anticipatory Struggle

Anticipatory struggle is a perspective on stuttering which differs considerably from many other perspectives considered in this section; it is a perspective which deals with the cause of the disorder. A causal theory about a disorder can be a statement of the physiological or medical reasons for its existence. Freeman and Usijima (1978) refer to such ultimate aberrations as distal causes. However, there is another type of causal explanation of stuttering, which is directed simply at explaining why stuttering occurs when someone attempts to speak. What happens to cause those day-to-day blocks, prolongations and repetitions? Freeman and Usijima refer to this as the proximal cause of stuttering. Distal and proximal explanations can be different, but equally important in understanding a disorder. For example, the proximal causes of asthma—exercise, food allergies, and so on—are different from whatever distal cause or causes might be responsible for someone having the condition.

There is no generally accepted explanation for the distal cause or causes of stuttering. In other words, the fundamental problem with people who stutter is unknown. However, the most influential speculation about the matter has come from a group of ideas which Bloodstein (1987) terms anticipatory struggle theory. Anticipatory struggle theory embraces Johnson's diagnosogenic theory, and various developments from that position which are popular among clinicians today. These theories have in common that people stutter because they believe that speech is difficult, and that this unhealthy belief system arises from pressures on speech and communication in the early years of life. This line of reasoning is explored below, and in Part Seven its relevance to clinical practice is explored.

## The theory of primary and secondary stuttering

Although Bluemel (1932) is generally credited with this theory, Bloodstein (1986) notes that similar ideas had been expressed by Froeschels (1915; 1933). The theory of primary and secondary stuttering is commonly thought of as an antecedent to the diagnosogenic theory. Effortless, unconscious repetitions were considered to be a common feature of the speech development of children, which would disappear in time if attention was not drawn to them. These repetitions were labelled "primary stutters." It was thought that the features of the so-called "secondary stuttering"—blocks, fear, embarrassment, and so on—would develop if the child was made apprehensive about the primary speech disruptions. "Secondary stuttering" was the name given to the fully developed stuttering syndrome. The terms "primary" and "secondary" stuttering are still used today by some clinicians.

## The diagnosogenic theory

Johnson was one of Travis' students at the University of Iowa during the first part of this century. In effect, Johnson (1942) added some sophistication to Bluemel's theory and gave it widespread popularity. He developed a theory that stuttering is caused when parents diagnose that their children are stuttering when, in fact, their children have normal disfluency. The diagnosogenic theory was discussed in Part Two, so a review of that material might be helpful before proceeding. The theory concerns the distal origins of stuttering, and that fact, combined with its simplicity, probably explains why it has been the most influential of all theories about stuttering. Perhaps another factor which contributed to the extensive influence of the diagnosogenic theory was that its fundamental premise was difficult to refute. This is because Johnson asserted that the child's speech is normal *at the time the diagnosis of stuttering is made by the parent*. It is virtually impossible for researchers to be present and collect speech data on a child at the precise moment that parents come to believe that the child has begun to stutter. By contrast, the Orton-Travis theory (see above) was easy to test by assessing the laterality of people who stutter, and it was quite short-lived because people who stutter did not have atypical laterality.

The declining credibility of the diagnosogenic theory in recent years (Bloodstein, 1986; 1987) may be due in part to the influence of behaviorism on stuttering management practices in the middle years of this century. As discussed previously, behavioral management of stuttering focuses on measurable behaviors in the planning, conduct and evaluation of treatments. Perhaps that doctrine counteracted the influence of Johnson's theory, which focused on the origins of the disorder. The behavioral reports of Martin, Kuhl, and Haroldson (1972) and Reed and Godden (1977) directly challenged the theory by showing that calling attention to a child's stuttering improved, not worsened, the condition (see page 119).

One of Johnson's own studies (reported in Johnson & Associates, 1959) contributed to the eventual downfall of his theory. This was a study of parents' recall of their children's speech when stuttering was thought to begin. Results showed that parents recalled distinctive speech features associated with the children thought to be stuttering; sound and syllable repetitions and sound prolongations. These speech features were not recalled as prominently by parents of nonstuttering children. These findings questioned Johnson's contention that at the time of diagnosis the speech of stuttering children was completely normal. Johnson's data for the above speech features, and others, showed considerable "overlap" between stuttering children and nonstuttering children. There was no feature which was not present—at least to a slight extent—in the speech of both groups. Johnson felt that these findings did not justify an abandonment of the theory that there was no essential difference between stuttering and nonstuttering children at the time of diagnosis of stuttering. He developed a more sophisticated statement of the premise that stuttering is induced by listener diagnosis. This was a "general interaction hypothesis" (Johnson & associates, 1959, Ch. 10), which still maintained the premise that stuttering was essentially a problem for the listener, not the speaker. This restatement of the theory implicated an interaction between several variables; the listener's readiness to perceive the speaker's "nonfluency" and to evaluate it negatively, the actual extent to which the speaker really is "nonfluent," and the extent of the speaker's own reaction to "nonfluent" speech, and the extent of the speaker's reaction to the reaction of others. However, this revised version of the diagnosogenic theory lost the engaging simplicity of the original idea which, arguably, was an important factor in its original success.

A prediction of the diagnosogenic theory is that stuttering would not exist in a culture where there was little pressure for children to develop verbal skills and where there was no word to describe the condition. Arguably, much of the theory's credibility once rested on Johnson's contention, based on anthropological surveys, that American Indians had no word for stuttering and that none of them experienced it. However Bloodstein (1987) lists as one of the most significant revelations about the disorder in recent times that "American Indians of the great plains do stutter and probably did stutter a generation ago, when they were reported not to." In quite a controversial report (see the reply by Stewart, 1985), Zimmermann, Liljeblad, Frank, and Cleeland (1983) presented their observations of two decades earlier that American tribes had both stuttering members and words for the condition. This report is corroborated by Van Riper (1971), who lists various tribal Indian words for stuttering, and by a report by Lemert (1953) that Indians stuttered and referred to the condition.

## The tension and fragmentation hypothesis

Bloodstein was a student of Johnson's who eventually became discontented with the diagnosogenic theory and developed the "tension and fragmentation hypothesis" (Bloodstein, 1986). This hypothesis has in common with Johnson's theory that it concerns anticipatory struggle; it focuses on early pressures which impact on speech and communication. The hypothesis presents a detailed explanation of the proximal cause of stuttering. According to Bloodstein (1987), day-to-day stuttering occurs because of a feeling of impending difficulty in speech which disrupts speech motor planning and execution;

> all of the integral features of stuttering behavior are reducible to the surface effects of two underlying forms of behavior—tension and fragmentation. Whenever we are faced with the threat of failure in the performance of a complex activity demanding accuracy or skill we are likely to make use of abnormal muscular tension. We are also apt to produce a portion of the act separately and sometimes repeatedly before we complete it. In stuttering the underlying tension produces prolongations and hard attacks. The repetitions of stuttering may be interpreted as a fragmentation of speech units somewhat analagous to the behavior of dart-throwers rehearsing the initial part of their throw. p. 53)

As a distal explanation, Bloodstein states that this form of anticipatory struggle

> develops readily in circumstances in which speech pressures are unusually heavy, the child's vulnerability to them unusually high, or the provocations in the form of communicative difficulties or failures unusually frequent, severe, or chronic. (pp. 366-367)

The most direct application of the tension and fragmentation hypothesis in clinical practice is outlined by Prins (1983). That program recommends identification and elimination of various kinds of environmental stressors that influence speech and communication. To establish the need for treatment, the clinician determines whether signs of tension and fragmentation are in the child's speech. Signs of frustration are an important indicator of the need for intervention. It is interesting that this management system does not recommend a decision to intervene according to whether or not a child is thought to be stuttering. Instead, the decision to intervene is based on the presence or absence of factors thought to precipitate stuttering. Prins specifies several sources of pressures/stresses on the child that should be removed in treatment. For example,

> *General* sources of environmental stress and uncertainty: erratic planning and conduct of routine daily activities including meals and bedtime...continuing, unpredictable changes in the makeup of the "family" constellation, including relatives and visitors who sometimes live in the home, parental absences, etc.... insufficient time spent alone with the child and in attending to his individual needs.

and

> *Specific* sources of communicative pressure and uncertainty:...poor listening on the part of parents and family...parental speech characteristics that are complex, rushed, and impatient...a competitive speaking environment including—persistently—multiple speakers and listeners. (original italics) (Prins, 1983; p. 28)

# The "interactionist" view

An extension of anticipatory struggle theory is that stuttered speech does not reflect only the environmental influences on a child's speech, but an interaction between those influences and the child's physical capacity for speech. A paper by Andrews, Craig, Feyer, Hoddinott, Howie, and Neilson (1983) is an early source of this idea. Williams (1984) Conture (1982) and Conture and Caruso (1987) also have presented this "interactionist" view:

> stuttering relates to a complex interaction between the child's environment and the skills and abilities the child brings to that environment...That is, we believe that stuttering can best be considered and treated in terms of how the client's skills and abilities interact with his or her environment. (Conture & Caruso, 1987, p. 87)

Starkweather in effect has made similar statements with a "demands and capacities model" (Starkweather, 1987), where stutter-free speech in childhood is dependent on environmental demands on speech not exceeding the child's capacity for "fluent speech." The capacity for "fluent speech" is outlined in four categories; "speech motor control, language formulation, social-emotional maturity, and cognitive skill" (p. 14). There are recent signs that the demands and capacities model is gaining popularity. For example, Adams (1990) has discussed it, and Weiss and Zebrowski (1992) have tested its clinical implications.[1]

Starkweather and colleagues have outlined the clinical application of the demands and capacities model (Starkweather & Gottwald, 1990, Starkweather, Gottwald, & Halfond, 1990). Treatment procedures derived from it resemble the program by Prins (1983) outlined above, in the sense that certain features of the child's communicative environment are targeted for modification. Potential demands on fluency are outlined under categories of various time pressures and insecurities in the child's life, and various direct and indirect things that parents might do to convey to the child that stuttering is undesirable.

# Strengths and weaknesses of anticipatory struggle theory[2]

*Strengths of Explanatory Power.* As noted by Wingate (1983), knowledge and understanding are different things. Much is known about this disorder, and one function of causal theory should be to transform that knowledge into understanding by a process of explanation. Anticipatory struggle theory contributes much to the understanding of stuttering because it offers convincing explanations for some of the disorder's distinctive phenomenology (see Bloodstein, 1984).

Anticipatory struggle theory provides a credible explanation of the consistency and adjacency effects. The consistency effect is that stuttering tends to occur on the same words on repeated readings of the same passage. There is some evidence for a much more interesting effect called adjacency (see Bloodstein, 1987, for a review of research into these effects). If words on which a speaker stutters are removed from a passage, there seems to be a tendency for stuttering to occur on words which are close to the originally stuttered words. According to anticipatory struggle theory, these effects occur because words are representative of past speech failure and apprehension, and as such function as stimuli for speech breakdowns.

---

[1] The Weiss and Zebrowski (1992) study will be discussed in a later section.

[2] This section includes portions of Onslow (1992), which are reprinted by permission of the American Speech-Language-Hearing Association.

Another phenomenon, the adaptation effect (see Part One), can be explained in terms of lessening apprehension about speech as familiarity with read material increases. Bloodstein (1984) also argues that the predominance of stuttering on word initial sounds suggests that the disorder involves perceived difficulties with the speech process, rather than a general incapacity to produce the sounds of speech. Anticipatory struggle theory also explains the often reported fact that people who stutter have idiosyncratic speech difficulties of various kinds, and it explains the effects of audience size and speaking situation on stuttering.

*Shortcomings in Explanatory Power.* As is always the case with theories of the cause of stuttering, anticipatory struggle theory has some shortcomings in explanatory power. One shortcoming is the involvement of cognition in stuttering. Bloodstein (1984) has even gone as far as asserting that people would recover from the disorder immediately if they could forget that they stuttered. However, this is difficult to accept in light of the generally accepted conclusion that, alone, cognitive-based procedures such as hypnosis, anxiety reduction, and psychotherapy, are of limited value in eliminating stuttered speech.[1] If anticipatory struggle theory is to be tenable, such procedures should make a major contribution to the elimination of stuttered speech. It also is difficult to accept the cognitive bases of anticipatory struggle theory in the light of knowledge that stuttering can develop suddenly, in some cases in a single day (Onslow, Harrison, & Jones, 1993; Yairi, 1983).[2] Sudden onset is not a characteristic of human problems that involve negative emotion. Normally, there is a protracted history of such problems, including progressive worsening.

Another serious challenge to the tenability of anticipatory struggle theories arises from the role of anxiety in stuttering. If those theories were tenable, then anxiety would be expected to be an integral component of the disorder: A relationship between anxiety and stuttering would yield readily to empirical scrutiny and assume a place among the few undisputed facts about the disorder. However, as considered in a later section, it is far from clear that there is a link between stuttering and anxiety. This is especially problematic considering that most of the explanatory power of anticipatory struggle theory rests on its capacity to account for the disorder in terms of apprehension about speech.

There is a further serious limitation of the explanatory power of anticipatory struggle theory. As discussed previously, one of the few undisputed facts about the disorder is that genetics plays some role in its development, although genetic explanations appear not to be able to account for all occurrences of stuttering. Bloodstein (1984; 1987) has focussed on the incompleteness of genetic explanations in arguing that environmental factors might be implicated in stuttering. As mentioned previously, one role of an etiological theory about stuttering should be to provide understanding through explanation of available knowledge. However, Bloodstein's arguments provide no such understanding of genetic material, but state merely that genetic and environmental influences can coexist. Bloodstein recognizes this problem:

> On the whole, our hypothesis does not as readily account for the familial incidence of stuttering or other evidence of possible genetic influences. While the theory can be reconciled with such facts by various means, it does not afford any special insight into them, and we are left in doubt as to their precise meaning. (1987, p. 367)

---

[1] This comment should not be taken as a suggestion that such procedures are unnecessary in the management of stuttering. On the contrary, some cognitively-based procedures, such as counselling, are indispensible in management of the disorder, but are not useful as primary means to eliminate stuttered speech.

[2] The author has encountered one case of early stuttering that was referred from a hospital casualty department.

Bloodstein (1987) also acknowledges a further problem with using the incompleteness of genetic explanations of stuttering as support for anticipatory struggle. It is true that genetic research has determined that nongenetic factors play a role in the development of stuttering. However, nongenetic factors are not necessarily the environmental factors of learning and cognition that comprise the anticipatory struggle theory. Random factors also contribute to the development of an organism (Kidd, 1984), and there are many random influences in nature that can be responsible for disorders, but which are independent of learning and cognition. For example, encephalitis is neither genetically transmitted nor learned. In order to establish whether the nongenetic factors associated with stuttering include communicative pressures, convincing empirical evidence needs to be brought forward. The following section draws attention to the fact that this has not occurred.

*Absence of empirical support.* Bloodstein (1984) uses a number of lines of indirect evidence in support of anticipatory struggle theory. It is argued that certain anthropological findings suggest that "there are cultural influences in the incidence of the disorder" (Bloodstein, 1987, p. 119). For example "stuttering tends to flourish in cultures that impose heavy competitive pressures for achievement and conformity." (p. 173). Further, Bloodstein supports the role of the environment by referring to

> a widespread impression among American clinical workers of long experience that the prevalence of stuttering is considerably less than it was some decades ago. (p. 123)

Bloodstein argues that a variety of environmental influences may be responsible for this decreasing prevalence, including social changes in child rearing practices and the influence of the diagnosogenic theory. It is also suggested that the recent establishment of the speech-language pathology profession may have been influential in spurring a change in the attitudes in society toward those who stutter. Overall, Bloodstein concludes that

> the environmental factor to which a probably causal relationship can be most clearly discerned in studies of the incidence of stuttering in various populations is competitive pressure for achievement or conformity (1987; p. 355)

The important implications of anticipatory struggle theory for stuttering management compel a careful consideration of Bloodstein's arguments. Bloodstein (1987) himself acknowledges that anthropological evidence concerning cultural influences on stuttering is "fragmentary" (p. 119). Even stronger doubts have been voiced by Van Riper (1971), who commented that prevalence and incidence data for non-Western cultures "is appallingly meager and its validity seems questionable" (p. 41). To that should be added that the coexistence of (a) low stuttering rates and (b) "low competitive pressures for achievement and conformity" cannot be be interpreted as support for a causal relation between the two. With regard to the claim of lessening prevalence of stuttering in recent years, again Bloodstein expresses doubts. He states that there is "little adequate evidence on the question" (Bloodstein, 1987, p. 123). In any event, as noted by Van Riper (1971), if fewer clients who stutter are presenting for treatment than in the past, then that is a statement of clinical trends, and should not be taken as an epidemiological statement. At the very least, Bloodstein's (1987) claim that falling prevalence of the disorder is "one of the strongest indications that can be found of the contribution of the environment to the etiology of stuttering" (p. 123) should be seriously challenged.

The citing of indirect evidence for anticipatory struggle theory underscores the current lack of direct evidence for the theory. Martin and Haroldson (1986) have suggested that one assessment of the contribution of a theory is the number of empirical research questions it is capable of generating. But as noted previously, the central premises of anticipatory struggle theories are resistant to verification. The tension and fragmentation hypothesis would be directly verified by an assessment of "speech pressures" and "communicative difficulties or failures" (Bloodstein, 1987, pp. 366-367) in the families of incipient stuttering children, along with an assessment of those children's "vulnerability to them". (p. 366) However, the lack of any detail about the nature of those causative agents precludes scientific investigation of them with testable hypotheses. A further avenue to verify anticipatory struggle theory is unavailable because ethical considerations prevent experiments where normally speaking children would be subjected to the environments that are thought to cause stuttering.

## Anticipatory struggle theory: Final comments

The above sections have considered the extensive contribution of Johnson and Bloodstein in theorizing about the onset of stuttering and how it should be treated in early childhood. The section would not be complete without mention of the contribution of the early Iowa clinicians to the treatment of adults. Bloodstein (1987) describes how in the 1930s Bryng Bryngelson, Wendell Johnson, and Charles Van Riper overrode the popular organic models of the day (see pages 124-125) in their thinking. Their clinical practices had in common that they combatted anticipatory struggle reactions by encouraging their adult clients to avoid hiding, fearing, or being ashamed of their stuttering. Van Riper has achieved revered status as a clinician. His therapeutic approach is grounded in the notions of anticipatory struggle to the extent that the point of treatment is not to "recover" from stuttering but to modify the speaker's response to stuttering. That modification involves teaching the client not to struggle with stuttering but to stutter in an effortless manner. This is often called the "stutter more fluently" approach. A preliminary part of Van Riper's treatment is to show the client the idiosyncratic way that stuttering is exacerbated by struggling with it. Van Riper's techniques for stuttering effortlessly are known as "cancellations," "preparatory sets," and "pull-outs."

There is no doubt that anticipatory struggle theories have had more collective impact on thinking about stuttering, and its clinical management, than any other view of its cause. There are several reasons that might explain such enduring popularity. Perhaps the original popularity of the diagnosogenic theory was responsible to some extent. For, although modern reiterations of anticipatory struggle are different from Johnson's, they still retain the role of a child's environment as a contributing factor in the development of stuttering. Anticipatory struggle also makes it easy to conceptualize the nature of the disorder. Arguably, this has been attractive to clinicians because, as mentioned previously, theoretical perspectives give clinicians a way to explain the condition to clients, and to explain why a recommended treatment might work. A final explanation for the continuing popularity of anticipatory struggle theories is that they have generally been resistant to either empirical verification or disproof. It is not surprising that a simple, understandable and clinically relevant idea such as anticipatory struggle has persisted if there has been no experimental evidence to challenge it.

# Learning

Several causal theories of stuttering have specifically incorporated learning theory approaches to human functioning and human problems. This section overviews three such learning theory approaches which have been used to present distal and proximal causes of stuttering.

## Instrumental[1] avoidance theory

There is an often-cited problem with the notion that learning is involved with stuttering: How can it be that stuttering persists when it attracts what must be powerful punishing social stimuli, and what can the reinforcer be that enables it to persist for a lifetime? Wischner (1950; 1952) attempted to answer such questions using the model of instrumental avoidance, and this was the first popular application of a learning theory to the problem of stuttering.

Instrumental avoidance conditioning involves presentation of a signal which indicates that a noxious stimulus is about to occur. If a certain response occurs shortly after the signal, then the noxious stimulus is avoided. With this type of learning, an animal will avoid shock by running in an apparatus in response to the sound of a signal such as a buzzer. It is presumed that the response is maintained by negative reinforcement through fear reduction. In other words, the running is a reinforcement because it removes the fear of the shock.

Instrumental avoidance has some appeal as an explanation for stuttering because this type of conditioning is notoriously resistant to extinction; the animal will not stop running even though the shock no longer occurs. This might be a way to explain why people who stutter continue to do so throughout their lives. However, in order to be tenable for stuttering, such a learning model requires a source of anxiety from which to escape. Wischner concurred with Johnson (see above) in suggesting that the source of such anxiety was parental disapproval of normal disfluencies and subsequent pressure. However, as pointed out by Van Riper (1971), Wischer's view differed from Johnson's in that it was the *anxiety* from which escape was sought; in Johnson's view it was the normal disfluencies that the child sought to avoid. In essence, Wischner speculated that stuttering is a disorder characterized by speech anxiety, and that stuttered speech is an avoidance reaction which is positively reinforced because it provides relief from that anxiety.

## Approach-avoidance theory

Another theory concerning avoidance was presented by Joseph Sheehan, who suggested that stuttered speech is the result of conflict between the desire to speak and the desire to avoid speaking.[2] This theory was derived from the results of animal research concerning

---

[1] The terms "instrumental" and "operant" can be loosely interchanged, although the latter term is normally applied in atheoretical analyses of behavior used originally by Skinner.

[2] Sheehan was a student of Johnson and Van Riper, and the influence of the Iowa school on his work is obvious. Sheehan's contribution is the only widely known formal theoretical statement about

approach-avoidance conflict (Miller, 1944). This research placed animals in a situation where they simultaneously experienced a drive to obtain food and a drive to avoid a shock. Animals were shown to vacillate in a region where the drive to approach food appeared to equal the drive to avoid shock. According to Sheehan, the repetitions and prolongations of stuttering are similar fixations at the point where the drives to speak and to avoid speaking are equal. In fact, Sheehan suggests that stuttering is a "double approach-avoidance conflict," with conflicting urges both to speak and to remain silent. This explanation of how stuttering occurs is accompanied by an explanation of how the person who stutters is able to proceed with speech when this fixation occurs; the stuttering moment reduces the fear that caused it, allowing the speaker to continue. Stuttering features other than the basic repetitions and prolongations are operant escape and avoidance behaviors. The theory states that the successful execution of these behaviors perpetuates the disorder.

Sheehan's major contention is that, although the basic conflict of stuttering is reflected at the word level, it is a disorder of personality, with conflicts at many levels of personal functioning, such as word level, situation level, emotional expression, relationships, self role (the latter refers to acceptance or rejection of role expectations). A recurring theme through Sheehan's writings is that, at the "deeper" levels of the disorder, stuttering characteristically involves guilt, fear, and shame; feelings that are suppressed along with avoidance and suppression of stuttered words. Sheehan's proximal explanation of stuttered speech as a manifestation of approach-avoidance conflicts is quite credible. However, a distal explanation of stuttering in similar terms seems tenuous by comparison; that stuttering develops through conflicts at the self-role level.

Sheehan posits that the perpetuation of stuttering is due to avoidance procedures used by the speaker, hence treatments derived from approach-avoidance theory are based on avoidance reduction. It is clear that there is no place in such a treatment for a concept that stuttered speech should be eliminated:

1. Your stuttering is a conflict between going ahead and holding back. To improve, you must reduce and finally get rid of the holding back of your habits of hiding and avoidance.
2. Your stuttering is a false-role disorder. You will remain a stutterer as long as you continue to pretend not to be one.
3. Just as you have stuttered most of your life up to now, you will stutter somewhat the rest of your life.
4. You have a choice as to *how* you stutter. You do not have a choice as to *whether* you stutter.
5. What you call your stuttering consists mostly of the tricks, the crutches you use to cover up. (Sheehan, 1975; p. 157)

Sheehan's treatment procedures for children are based on rectifying what he refers to as an imbalance in the "demand-support" ratio; the extent of the demands placed on the child in comparison to the support given to the child in attempts to meet those demands. In this regard, Sheehan's background at the University of Iowa seems to be discernible, because the onset of stuttering is regarded as a direct reflection of parenting:

> In situations where parents seem unwilling to change their ways, sometimes a visit to an adult stutterers' group will have a sobering effect. From behind the observation mirror, we may say something like this: "See that fellow over there with a grotesque grimace? Unless you stop picking at your son and help him to feel

---

stuttering as struggle in adulthood, and it might easily have been categorized as an anticipatory struggle theory.

more secure about himself, he's going to grow up to be like that." (Sheehan, 1975, p. 181)

# Two-factor theory

Classical conditioning involves stimuli that once were neutral, but which come to evoke a reflexive response. Operant conditioning involves voluntary responses that are not directly precipitated by stimuli, but relate in systematic ways to stimuli in the form of environmental events. Brutten and Shoemaker (1967) presented the idea that stuttering behaviors are two such classes of behavior, rather than one. It was theorized that repetitions and prolongations ("first factor responses") are classically conditioned, meaning that they are reflexive responses. All other stuttering events ("second factor responses") were thought be operantly conditioned avoidance responses. In other words, stuttering is a classically conditioned disorder, with avoidance responses operantly conditioned (word avoiding, interjecting, twitching, etc.).

Brutten and Shoemaker contend that negative emotional responses disrupt the cognitive and motor processes involved in speech, and these disruptions are the bases for the formation of "factor one" elements of stuttering in the early years of life: The relationship between the eliciting stimuli and emotional responses causes classically conditioned speech disruptions. Neutral stimuli associated with speech become conditioned stimuli through early speech experiences. Thus, "primary stutters" are nothing more than negative emotion which disrupts speech. All other stuttering features are avoidance.

There have been some challenges to two-factor theory. As Ingham (1984) points out, the reasoning behind the theory means that stuttering really is anxiety. In the absence of negative emotion, no speech events can be considered to be stuttering, regardless of how similar they may seem to stuttering. Yet, as considered in the next section, stuttering does not seem to be related to anxiety in such a clearly systematic way. Another challenge to two-factor theory comes from a study by Costello and Hurst (1981), who showed that when one type of stuttering event is reduced in frequency when punished, other stuttering events reduce also (see also Brutten, 1983; Costello & Hurst, 1981). This result is consistent with a view of stuttering as a unitary disorder, not a disorder involving more than one class of behavior.

# Anxiety[1]

## Research into stuttering and anxiety

Trait anxiety refers to a person's inherent level of anxiety, and state anxiety refers to condition- or situation-specific anxiety. As discussed previously, many theorists have implicated anxiety in the cause or the nature of stuttering (e.g. Bloodstein, 1987; Brutten & Shoemaker, 1967; Johnson, 1942; Sheehan, 1975; Travis, 1971; Wischner, 1950). So, if there is a substantive relation between stuttering and anxiety, then people who stutter should characteristically be more anxious than those who do not stutter, and should show elevated anxiety levels in certain speech situations. This proposition has been the topic of a considerable body of research.

In the 1980s several scholars reviewed research concerning stuttering and anxiety and agreed in their conclusions that little scientific evidence had been found for a systematic and predictable relationship between anxiety and stuttering. Andrews, Craig, Feyer, Hoddinott, Howie & Neilson (1983) concluded that

> there was considerable evidence collected about stutterers' personality attributes and their propensity to show anxiety or neurotic symptoms. No differences in personality factors related to neuroticism have been demonstrated in controlled studies of unselected populations (p. 229)

and Ingham (1984) concluded that

> the overall tenor of the findings from the studies reviewed is that there is little evidence of a clinically significant, or even theoretically palpable, relationship between stuttering and anxiety...Stutterers may appear to be anxious, even fearful, with respect to speaking situations, but it seems unlikely that variations in their speech problem are directly related to this fear or anxiety. (pp. 132-133)

and Bloodstein (1987) concluded that

> all we can say is that by the definitions of anxiety that are usual in clinical and experimental work, anxiety about stuttering has a distinct but inconsistent, limited, and qualified relationship to stuttering. (p. 287)

Since the time of those reviews there have been several important reports concerning stuttering and anxiety. From a clinical perspective, perhaps the most important of these has been Craig's (1990) study of anxiety in adults who were treated for stuttering. In formulating this study, Craig acknowledged that previous research consistently showed no relation between stuttering and anxiety, and reiterated the existing viewpoint that there is no available evidence of a causal relation between stuttering and anxiety. However, Craig noted that existing studies had low statistical power[2] because of small subject numbers, and hence they may have overlooked a functional relationship between stuttering and anxiety. Hence, the purpose of Craig's study was to search for such a relationship with a large sample size.

Subjects were 102 stuttering clients who were treated with an intensive treatment based on prolonged speech, and 102 control subjects who did not stutter. The treatment program

---

[1] This section was written with the assistance of Michelle Lincoln.

[2] Statistical power refers to how likely an analysis is to detect an effect if one is present. The higher the power of the analysis, the more chance the experimenters have of detecting an effect.

reduced the stuttering of the clients to a mean of less than 1 %SS within the clinic. Experimental subjects made a 5-minute telephone call to a stranger before treatment and after treatment, and controls made telephone calls at corresponding time intervals. After the phone call, each subject completed a questionnaire for assessing state and trait anxiety. The state anxiety measure was collected before treatment, but not after treatment. Forty-three of the 102 stuttering subjects completed the trait anxiety questionnaire after treatment. Results showed that state anxiety measures were significantly higher for the experimental group than measures for the controls after the pretreatment phone call. The stuttering subjects also showed significantly higher pretreatment trait anxiety than did controls. Craig concluded that "before treatment, the stutterers were shown to be more highly anxious on both state and trait measures than their fluent controls" (p. 292) and that "stutterers are more highly anxious as a group" (p. 293). Additionally the 43 clients who were measured for posttreatment trait anxiety achieved scores that were not significantly different from the control group.

There are some problems which weaken the external validity of the Craig study.[1] One problem is that the state anxiety measures pertained to the stuttering subjects' experience of speaking to a stranger on the telephone, so the interpretation of the results of the study pertain only to that speaking situation. As Craig comments, people who stutter seem to find the telephone particularly troubling, so the state anxiety assessment in the study could have been a particularly anxiety-provoking situation. Another external validity issue in the study is that subjects were clients in a specialist intensive treatment program and hence were not selected randomly. Because of this, the statistical analyses of the study were questionable (Attanasio, 1991; Craig, 1991). Further, the specialist nature of the treatment invokes concerns about the extent to which the anxiety of clients resembles the anxiety of those who stutter and who seek treatment in general. In a recent overview of this treatment program, Mooney (1990) reported that

> people have to be highly motivated to take part in the intensive course. The typical patient is…in his mid to late twenties with a moderately successful to very success-ful career. He is usually either facing a promotional block or has reached it. (p. 26)

Possibly, then, the group of subjects in the Craig report may have been atypical in terms of their motivation to eliminate stuttered speech. It is also possible that such a need to eliminate stuttering would be driven by anxiety about speech, particularly in cases where the seeking of treatment is driven by career pressures. This possibility considerably lessens the confidence that can be placed in Craig's findings of elevated pretreatment state and trait anxiety levels in the subjects studied. Those findings could have been due in part, or even completely, to the client selection biases of the program.

These uncertainties about Craig's results are substantiated by a more recent report by Miller and Watson (1992) which used the same questionnaire measures of anxiety as the former report but applied them to a more randomly chosen group of 52 people who stutter. Miller and Watson found no difference between a stuttering and control group in either state or trait anxiety scores. Kraaimaat, Janssen and Van Dam-Baggen (1991) reported a positive result when they compared levels of social anxiety among people who stutter, "social phobic" patients, and controls. They found that people who stutter were significantly more anxious than normal subjects but significantly less anxious than the social phobics.

Kraaimaat, Jansseen and Brutten (1988) found reductions in cognitive and some autonomic measures of anxiety after stuttering treatment in 33 adolescents. However, one inconsistency in this report was that a significant difference was found with only one of

---

[1] External validity is the extent to which general statements can be made from the results of research.

three autonomic measures. Weber and Smith (1990) measured skin conductance, peripheral blood flow and heart rate of subjects who stuttered and controls during speech and non-speech activities. They reported that both groups had similar levels of autonomic arousal during all activities. This finding is consistent with an earlier study by Peters and Hulstijn (1984). However in the Weber and Smith study, "disfluent" utterances in the subjects who stuttered were not associated with higher autonomic arousal than controls. Nonetheless, when comparing the stutterers' fluent utterances with their disfluent utterances, Weber and Smith found that higher autonomic levels correlated with disfluent speech. One problem with interpreting these results as an indicator of a relation between anxiety and stuttering is that all measures for both groups were within the normal range.

Lincoln and Onslow (1993) attempted to contribute information to the issue of stuttering and anxiety by surveying beliefs on the matter held by different groups of people; clinicians, people who stutter, and controls. They found that the majority of clinicians and people who stutter believed that anxiety is involved in the disorder (97 percent and 87 percent respectively), and that around two-thirds of clinicians reported regularly including anxiety management in their treatment of adult clients who stutter. However, respondents generally indicated that they believed state anxiety, not trait anxiety, to be the prominent form of anxiety in stuttering. Comparisons of self-reported anxiety between people who stutter and a control group were consistent with this result, with markedly more stuttering subjects reporting that they "frequently" experienced speech-related state anxiety.

The Lincoln and Onslow data suggested that people who stutter are not a homogeneous group in their experiences of anxiety: 31 percent of stuttering respondents reported that they experienced neither trait nor speech-related state anxiety, and, in a different part of the survey, 41 percent of them reported that they were anxious about speaking only "sometimes," and 21 percent of them reported such anxiety "rarely." Lincoln and Onslow suggested that these results might explain why researchers have not found a clear relation between anxiety and stuttering. Simply, anxiety associated with the disorder may be predominantly state anxiety about speaking. In which case, more studies such as Craig's (1990) are needed to explore the anxiety of people who stutter as they speak in situations in which anxiety is likely to occur.

## Clinical scenarios with stuttering and anxiety

In summary, the preceding overview shows that researchers have not convincingly demonstrated the existence of a link between stuttering and anxiety. To a clinician though, that situation is probably of limited interest because it is obvious that someone who stutters may experience anxiety and need their treatment adapted accordingly. Arguably it is also obvious that anxiety is not likely to be a problem with all people who stutter, as the results of Lincoln and Onslow (1993) confirm. Hence, routine inclusion of anxiety management procedures in stuttering treatments is likely to waste clinical resources. In the following, some clinical scenarios concerning stuttering and anxiety are considered.

*Anxiety is not a clinical issue.* This is a case of stuttering where anxiety seems not to be an issue. The client neither complains of anxiety, nor relates any history of trait or speech-related anxiety, nor shows any clinical signs of anxiety. Further, no signs of anxiety emerge during the course of treatment. The client learns stutter-free speech and then uses that stutter-free speech in conversational situations in which stuttering previously occurred. Such a client may even enter speaking situations which previously were avoided, not because of anxiety, but because communication in those situations was difficult. With such clients it is important to keep in mind that, at some stage, everyone is likely to experience speech-related anxiety in situations such as talking to a group or being interviewed. So the clinician needs to have some idea of how much speech anxiety a person would encounter in everyday life, and how much is clinically significant. It is not realistic to expect stuttering clients to be free of speech-related anxiety at all times.

*Anxiety is the presenting problem.* Clients exist whose fundamental complaint is that they are anxious. Most typically, these clients complain of debilitating speech anxiety about certain speaking situations; so much so that they either avoid those situations completely or enter them at the cost of an anxiety attack. Speaking on the telephone is notorious for posing such serious problems for people who stutter. As discussed in Part Two, the complaints of the client should be what drive clinical practice, so it would be an error to treat such a client with a program designed to eliminate stuttered speech. Such clients may only wish to be able to deal with their anxiety and may not particularly care about eliminating stuttered speech. Cases where clients stutter but also suffer from emotional problems involving trait anxiety can present quite a confusing picture to the clinician. This is because such clients can mistakenly link anxiety to stuttering.[1] It is easy for clients who have emotional problems to make a misjudgement that their anxiety problems are related to their stuttering when they really have more global problems.

*Stuttering eliminated but anxiety remains.* It may occur that a treatment program removes stuttered speech but this does not result in the elimination of speech-related anxiety. It might be argued that this is a clinical scenario that should not be allowed to happen, because once procedures to establish and generalize stutter-free speech have been concluded, clinical opportunities to help the client overcome speech-related anxiety have been lost. Those who subscribe to this viewpoint maintain that the best way to manage such clients is to specifically alter the treatment so that the learning of stutter-free speech is combined with anxiety management. It is not the best strategy to wait until it becomes clear that anxiety is persisting and then introduce anxiety management strategies. So, according to this viewpoint, the best management for clients with speech anxiety is to routinely incorporate anxiety management strategies within the treatment program. The opposing viewpoint is that management of stuttered speech and speech anxiety can occur independently, hence it is best to withhold anxiety management until it becomes clear that there is posttreatment speech anxiety.

*Anxiety eliminated with stuttered speech.* This clinical scenario is that the client presents with anxiety which resolves with the acquisition of stutter-free speech. In other words, the client's anxiety is due entirely to stuttered speech, and that anxiety ceases to exist when stuttered speech is not present. Some clinicians might argue that this would occur only with mild cases of speech-related anxiety, and that it is not likely that clinically significant anxiety would cease to be a problem with the elimination of stuttered speech. Another issue to consider is whether the clinician should expect speech anxiety to resolve immediately after the acquisition of stutter-free speech, or whether a period of time should be allowed to elapse before deciding that anxiety persists as a clinical problem. However, this ceases to be an issue if the clinician takes the option considered above of incorporating anxiety management procedures into the treatment of all anxious clients.

*Anxiety becomes apparent during treatment.* Some people who stutter organize their lives around the limitations that their speech problem imposes on them. This may prevent the experience of anxiety because a client simply never enters speaking situations in which

---

[1] The same comment applies to many kinds of personal problems such as lack of confidence, depression, and social isolation. The things people with such conditions complain about can resemble the complaints of people who stutter.

anxiety is likely to occur. However, many treatments for stuttering, particularly intensive treatments based on prolonged speech (see Part Four), require that the client enters a variety of speaking situations after achieving stutter-free speech. If that part of the treatment introduces the client to speaking situations which have habitually been avoided, an anxiety reaction may occur. Effective management of such of a problem depends on the clinician becoming aware before treatment of the extent to which the client avoids speaking situations. With that information, measures can be made to assist the client in entering new situations with stutter-free speech.

# Part Six:

# Clinical Issues in Management of Advanced Stuttering

# How Effective are Prolonged-Speech Treatments?

In Part Five it was argued that clinicians can be confident in the value of a treatment if it can be justified from a theoretical perspective. From the perspective of speech motor control, there is no doubt that prolonged-speech treatments are justifiable. If stuttered speech is a problem with speech motor control, then an effective counter to that problem is to teach the client a way of speaking that keeps that problem in check. However, clinicians require more to be completely confident in a treatment. No matter how theoretically sound a treatment is, there is no point in using it if it doesn't work. Hence, there is much to be learned from soundly designed clinical trials which establish the extent to which a treatment might be expected to control stuttered speech.

Onslow and Ingham (1989) reported a survey concerning the use by Australian speech pathologists of intensive treatments based on prolonged speech. A 48.5% return rate provided a total of 86 interpretable responses, which showed that 969 people who stutter had been assessed in the previous year. Table 4 shows the portions of those clients, by age group, who were referred for treatment programs based on prolonged speech that was administered as "daily therapy over a prescribed period."

TABLE FOUR: Referrals for intensive treatment programs based on prolonged speech, adapted from Onslow and Ingham (1989).

|  | Total Treated | Treated With Intensive Prolonged Speech |
| --- | --- | --- |
| preschool (younger than 5 years) | 210 | 24% |
| child (6-12 years) | 184 | 35% |
| adolescent (13-18 years) | 129 | 60% |
| adult (older than 19 years) | 195 | 88% |

Table 4 substantiates an impression that intensive prolonged speech treatment is a popular procedure in Australia. Table 4 also shows that the popularity of the procedure seems to extend to the point where many clinicians have used it for preschool-age children. Considering this widespread popularity of intensive prolonged treatments, it is particularly important to evaluate its effectiveness. However, there are two major difficulties in assessing whether the popularity of prolonged speech is justified. First, there are numerous criteria which can be used to evaluate the outcome of prolonged speech treatments. Second, researchers and scholars disagree in their conclusions about the effectiveness of these treatments in eliminating stuttered speech. This section considers whether intensive prolonged-speech treatment is effective according to various criteria, and looks at reports of its effectiveness.

study to compare the effects of a prolonged speech treatment with a syllable-timed speech (see Part One) treatment. Assessments were based on 1,000 syllables of speech collected within the clinic at the following intervals; 6 months pretreatment, immediately pretreatment, immediately posttreatment, 3 months, 6 months and 9 months posttreatment. For 23 clients, percent syllables stuttered scores for these assessments were, respectively, 18.16, 16.41, 0.11, 1.80, 0.58, 0.50. In another part of the development of this program, Ingham (1980) studied nine clients who had just completed the Generalization Phase of the treatment. In this study, 1,300-syllable speech samples were collected at six intervals from 4 months posttreatment to 24 months posttreatment, and were collected from within and beyond-clinic speaking situations. The data showed that all speech measures for all subjects, within and beyond the clinic, were below 0.8 %SS in the 24-month period.

The Ingham (1980) study was designed to show the relative merits of programmed and nonprogrammed maintenance. The clients were divided into two groups; one group that received programmed maintenance and one group that received nonprogrammed maintenance. Clearly, the clients with programmed maintenance achieved better results.[1] A practical advantage of programmed maintenance is that clients consume clinical time according to their needs during the maintenance phase of their treatment. If they continue to meet their program targets, then they consume progressively less clinical time. In contrast, a maintenance schedule which is independent of client performance might expend much clinician effort on clients who do not need it to maintain their treatment targets.

Boberg and colleagues (Boberg, 1980; 1981; 1986; Boberg & Kully, 1985; Boberg & Sawyer, 1977) have developed a 3-week residential prolonged speech program which is conducted in Alberta, Canada. Boberg (1981) reported data for 16 clients in this program who were given a variation on Ingham's (1980) performance-contingent schedule, and six clients who did not receive a maintenance program. The 16 clients who received the performance-contingent maintenance were assessed at pretreatment, immediately post-treatment, and at 6 and 12 months follow up. Speech measures reported are "percent disfluency," which is equivalent to %SS. At each assessment occasion, 2 or 3 minutes of speech was recorded in four situations; being interviewed by a stranger outside the clinic, reading, a conversation with a stranger which the clients tape recorded, and a telephone conversation with a stranger. Mean percent disfluency scores for the group at the four assessment occasions, across assessment situations, were, respectively, 16.38 (range 3.80-46.31), 1.86 (range 0.29-6.69), 2.30 (range 0.64-6.13), and 2.54 (0.76-7.41).

The group that did not receive the maintenance program was assessed only in the first two speaking situations described above, and were assessed at 12-months and 24-months follow-up. Consequently, it is difficult to judge from these subjects' data whether their outcome was worse for not having the maintenance program. Also, data was available only for three subjects at each follow-up assessment. And the pretreatment percent disfluency scores of these subjects as a group were nearly double that of the other group, and their immediate posttreatment scores were higher. Nonetheless, the data at least suggested that absence of the maintenance program worsened outcome at the 12-month follow-up, with these subjects scoring a mean of 7.49 percent disfluency (range 1.30-13.60) compared to a mean of 2.30 in the group who received maintenance.

In many ways these data are more informative about treatment outcome than those reported for other programs. The mean scores can be interpreted better because they are accompanied by the scores for individual clients. Further, Boberg and colleagues' studies

---

[1] All subjects' stuttering rates were low in this study, and may reflect the benefits of any kind of regular clinician contact during the first two years posttreatment.

share with Ingham's studies (see above) the advantages that clients are assessed several times and in beyond-clinic speaking situations. Boberg and Kully also present details of how clinicians were trained to collect "percent dysfluency" measures. Also, care was taken not to imply that the residential phase of treatment was all that was needed to achieve the reported results. Boberg reported that many clients in the program attended for "refresher weekends" at least once during the follow-up period. So the outcome data reflect the results of those "refresher weekends" in addition to the residential program. The importance of this aspect of service provision is often overlooked. Many Australian programs require or strongly recommend that clients join a support group after their treatment. But as Ingham (1984) points out, as is evident in a later section, membership of that association is likely to involve much treatment during attendance at group meetings. In addition, the Australian Speak Easy Association organizes regular "booster" treatments for its members.

The most recent outcome data for the Boberg program are supplied in a treatment manual (Boberg & Kully, 1985). The outcome of seven clients are reported (all of whom attended for "refresher weekends"). Boberg and Kully state that these clients "illustrate typical performance" of clients in their program. Within-clinic, 3-minute pretreatment speech samples show a mean of 25.12 percent dysfluency (range 50.0-7.35), and 3-minute posttreatment samples collected at the conclusion of the 3-week residential program show a mean of 1.03 percent dysfluency (range 0-2.10). These clients were assessed also at posttreatment intervals of 4 months, 6 months, 8 months, 16 months, and 24 months. These data were based on telephone call enquiries made from within the clinic, consisting of 2 minutes of accumulated speaking time. Mean percent dysfluency scores were, respectively, 4.64 (range 10.80-1.30), 3.16 (range 1.45-4.94), 2.60 (0.57-3.08), 7.22 (range 1.87-22.5), and 3.89 (range 2.32-8.0). The clients appear not to have received the maintenance program described by Boberg (1981).

One problem with the measures in the Boberg and Kully report is that the pretreatment and immediately posttreatment data were collected by clinicians, but all the posttreatment data were based on average counts of stutters as judged by "six adults selected from the community" (p. 18). The rationale for this was to determine "how much of the clients' residual stutters would be noticed by people outside the clinic" (p. 18). This makes it difficult to compare the follow-up measures with the pretreatment and immediate posttreatment measures, especially since two different speaking tasks were involved.

## Conclusions

The reports outlined above appear to have satisfied only some of Bloodstein's criteria for determining whether a treatment is effective. They evaluated clients for periods of between 9 and 24 months, and it is a matter for some debate whether that constitutes the "long term follow-up investigations" called for by Bloodstein. They certainly are "based on objective measures of speech behavior such as frequency of stuttering or rate of speech" (Bloodstein, 1987, p. 401). Bloodstein also called for outcome evaluation to include beyond-clinic speaking situations, repeated evaluations and substantial speech samples. Only some of the reports above satisfied those requirements.[1]

---

[1] A report by James, Ricciardelli, and Rogers (1989) involved repeated assessments in several beyond-clinic settings with substantial speech samples. However, data were only reported for a 6-month posttreatment period, hence this study did not fit the criteria for a "comprehensive" assessment as described previously.

One particular problem in the studies cited above is that they probably did not measure speech which was free of association with the clinic. This is obviously the case for the within-clinic speech samples which appear in many studies. And although it is a methodological improvement, beyond-clinic speech samples may also have this problem. In the Ingham (1980) study, for example, data came from tape recordings made mostly with the knowledge of subjects, who presumably also knew the purpose of those recordings. With regard to telephone assessments, Ingham (1984) has noted that in Webster's (1980) report clinic staff telephoned the clients, and the Howie, Tanner, and Andrews' (1981) telephone assessments were conducted by a psychologist who mentioned the treatment program and discussed future assessment. Boberg and Kully's (1985) telephone assessments were made while the clients were in the clinic. In short, the results of studies may indicate the extent to which clients were capable of producing stutter-free speech, but it is debatable whether they indicate the extent to which clients actually did so during their everyday lives.

Considering that clients who are treated with prolonged speech may use an unnatural sounding speech pattern, it is concerning that these reports did not follow Bloodstein's suggestion that they determine how natural the clients sounded. As considered in a later section, clients in prolonged-speech programs are likely to achieve stuttering reductions at the expense of natural sounding speech. In which case, the stuttering reductions reported in the literature are far less impressive. This is especially the case considering that assessments were linked to the clinic. Under such conditions clients may be prepared to use speech which sounds unnatural. However, speaking in customary life situations is a different matter.

External validity is a factor which limits the value of these treatment reports. They convey only the results achieved in specialized facilities, which contain clinicians with specialized skills. It is unknown whether those reports communicate anything meaningful to generalist clinicians who seek to know how effective such programs might be if they attempt them with their clients. Another external validity issue in prolonged speech outcome research is the obvious selection biases of subjects in those reports. Obviously, clients who undertake the rigors of intensive treatment are unlikely to be representative of the typical client encountered by clinicians. As discussed on page 146, clients who enrol in intensive programs may be more motivated to succeed in treatment than those found in a generalist clinic caseload.

Some reports verify the suggestion that the effectiveness of prolonged speech treatments might suffer if they are removed from the facility where they were developed and are normally conducted. Mallard and Kelley (1982) presented a report of their adaptation of Webster's Precision Fluency Shaping progamme, in which clients obviously did not do as well at follow-up as clients in the original program. As part of an evaluation of posttreatment speech quality in a Dutch adaptation of Precision Fluency Shaping, Franken, Boves, Peters, and Webster (1992) obtained 45-second speech samples for perceptual analysis from 32 clients. Samples from 5-minute within-clinic recordings taken pretreatment, posttreatment, and at 6-months follow-up. Mean pretreatment, posttreatment and follow-up %SS scores were, respectively, 25.7, 5.8, and 16.3. Although this was a perceptual study rather than an outcome study, these data certainly suggest that the program did not control stuttering as effectively as the original. Indeed, a summary of the outcome results of this program, based on within-clinic %SS measures, confirms this suggestions (Franken, Peters, & Tettero, 1989).

Treatment "dropouts" is an issue raised by Bloodstein which is related to external validity. It is well known to clinicians that intensive prolonged speech treatment is not suitable for all clients, but for how many clients this is the case is not clear from the outcome literature. Some reports specify exactly how many clients dropped out. For example Boberg and Kully (1985) report that

> approximately 300 stutterers have enrolled in summer clinics and completed this program. They have come from all parts of Canada and have ranged in age from 13 to 61. Only three clients left before completing the three-week program. (p. 17)

However it is likely that so few dropouts occurred because of increased motivation of the clients who travelled to attend such a specialized clinic. Also, the skill of specialist clinicians in assessing the suitability of the treatment for individual clients may also contribute to a low dropout rate. Martin (1981) suggests that around one-third might be a realistic estimate of dropout rate. A report by Franck (1980) suggests that the figure might be higher if it includes generalist clinics which attempt to adapt their facilities for intensive prolonged speech treatments, and if it also includes the maintenance phase of treatment. Franck reported that only 124 of 441 clients (28 percent) completed the maintenance phase of a prolonged speech treatment program which was conducted in the speech pathology department of a public hospital. Additionally, the data presented by Boberg (1981; see above) show that 8 of 16 clients (50 percent) completed a 12-month maintenance program.

In summary, though, there is little doubt of the following. In the hands of specialist clinicians, variations of intensive prolonged-speech treatment are capable of providing some clients with the skill to eliminate most of their stuttered speech for as long as two years. That skill is at its peak as soon as the intensive part of the treatment finishes, and a little of it is lost over time. Continued contact with clinicians, in the form of maintenance activities and/or "booster" programs, or contact with a self-help group, will probably assist to maintain that skill. It is unknown to what extent clients have stutter-free, natural-sounding speech during everday life after an intensive prolonged speech treatment.

## Formulating a general statement

One function of clinical research is to establish general statements about the effectiveness of treatments. There is some disagreement about the general statement that should be made about the effectiveness of intensive prolonged speech treatments, and this has led to several exchanges in the literature (for example, Andrews & Craig, 1988; Craig, 1989; Finn & Gow, 1989; Ingham & Onslow, 1990). Andrews, Guitar, and Howie (1980) performed a statistical procedure called meta-analysis on data from available treatment reports. The results led those authors to conclude that prolonged speech treatments are more effective than other styles of treatment. This meta analysis, along with the results of their investigations of the Prince Henry treatment program, have led Andrews and colleagues to conclude that prolonged-speech treatments have short and long-term effectiveness (Craig, Feyer, and Andrews, 1987; Andrews & Howie, 1984):

> It is pleasing that a disorder which disables communication ability can be virtually eliminated by treatment in the short-term and maintained in the long-term for the majority of stutterers. (Craig, Feyer, & Andrews, 1987, pp.60)

A more cautious position was presented by Ingham (1984):

> In general terms, at least, it is probable that numerous subjects who have passed through these treatment programs have gained markedly improved speech that generalized to nonclinic situations over about 2 years. But their speech is not necessarily equatable with normal-sounding speech, and, in many instances, it is probably retained at the cost of constant attention to speech production. (pp. 371-372)

Martin (1981) reviewed treatment literature (which consisted mostly of prolonged speech treatments) and concluded with the following estimate:

> One-third of the clients achieved and maintained satisfactory fluency...one-third of the clients achieved satisfactory fluency during treatment but experienced significant regression over time...almost one-third of all clients studied either failed to complete a treatment program or were unavailable for subsequent follow-up assessment. (p. 16)

This view is supported by Boberg, Howie, and Woods (1979):

> In summary, we have reviewed evidence which suggests that virtually all forms of intensive behavioral treatment of stuttering produce immediate dramatic increases in fluency, but encounter serious relapse problems in the posttreatment environment. (p. 115)

What can clinicians make of all this research into prolonged speech treatment outcome, and the interpretations of it? It certainly would be a reckless step to believe that the matter was closed and prolonged-speech treatments are as effective as they can be. Perhaps the best approach is to leave room for questions. As Ingham and Onslow (1990) have suggested, clinicians' questions about the treatments they use are important because they encourage developments in those treatments. If there are no questions, there are not likely to be any treatment developments. The following section pursues some of the sources of questioning about this style of treatment.

# Conceptual and Practical Shortcomings of Prolonged-Speech Treatments[1]

There are some conceptual and practical limitations of prolonged speech treatment. It is worthwhile to recognize those limitations, because they may influence a decision about whether prolonged speech or an RCS-based treatment is suitable for a client. The purpose of this section is to explore those limitations. The section pertains mostly to intensive treatment formats, but much of it pertains to the general idea of replacing stuttered speech with prolonged speech.

## Commonsense

In several ways, the recent popularity of prolonged speech seems to have overridden "clinical commonsense." In the first place, the treatment depends on a speech pattern change, but it does not seem likely that all clients can be treated optimally with the same speech pattern. It is far more likely that different clients will respond better to speech patterns which are individually designed for them. Yet intensive prolonged speech programs teach clients the same speech pattern with target behaviors such as "easy phrase intitiation," "phrase continuity" "continuous vocalization," "continuous airflow," "soft contacts," and "gentle onsets," and so on. It seems rarely to have been suggested or researched that there might be value in attempting to determine for each client which of those target behaviors are the most useful. Further, it is obvious when listening to the speech patterns used in these treatments that they incorporate many acoustic changes. Yet there is no reason to believe that all those changes are necessary for effective control of stuttering. It is a logical possibility that all variants of prolonged speech have in common a small number of acoustic variables—or even one acoustic variable—which alone is sufficient to control stuttering. There is some convincing research which suggests this may be so. Ingham, Montgomery, and Ulliana (1983) showed that stuttering may be controlled merely by decreasing the number of short periods of phonation.[2] Or stuttering may be controlled by reducing variability during speech (Onslow, van Doorn, & Newman, 1992; Packman, Onslow, & van Doorn, in press; Packman, van Doorn, & Onslow, 1992). If a single speech variable can functionally control stuttering, then at present many clinical hours may be wasted in the teaching of unnecessary components of prolonged speech.

Another way intensive prolonged speech programs seem to have overridden clinical commonsense is by endorsing the practice of removing clients from everyday speaking situations and placing them in groups for long periods for the purpose of teaching stutter-free speech. In the case of residential treatment settings, this isolation continues day and night until stutter-free speech has been established. The aim of treatment is to eliminate

---

[1] This section is based on Onslow and Ingham (1989).

[2] This acoustic change may be one of those invoked when a clinician instructs a client in "continuous vocalization."

stuttering in everyday situations, but removing clients from such situations is hardly a justifiable way to achieve that aim. Ingham (1984) has made the interesting suggestion that group treatments were misguidedly modelled after the experimental groups in the early Australian experiments with prolonged speech, although those experiments were not meant to imply that a group setting was a suitable model for treatment provision.

With all this in mind it is hard to overlook the benefits of a nonintensive approach to the teaching of prolonged speech. Once- or twice-weekly visits to a clinic would provide opportunities for the client to integrate a new speech pattern into customary speaking environments as the treatment progresses. In the case of school-age children, removal from normal speaking environments is a particular problem. Children obviously depend on the support of parents for success in maintaining stutter-free speech. But more importantly, the success of a child's treatment depends on parental instruction. It is difficult to imagine that a child's treatment could be effective if parents do not learn the features of prolonged speech and learn also to monitor their children's use of this pattern. Therefore, isolating parents from a prolonged speech treatment program probably inhibits their involvement at this level in their children's rehabilitation. Turnbaugh and Guitar (1981) provide a case study which shows how nonintensive prolonged speech treatment might be implemented with a child.

James, Ricciardelli, Rogers, and Hunter (1989) conducted an experiment to assess whether an intensive prolonged-speech treatment produced better results than a nonintensive version of the same program. A group of 11 clients were treated for 8 hours each day for 4 days (four 2-hour sessions each day) and another group of nine clients were treated with two 2-hour sessions each week for 8 weeks. This meant that both groups received 32 hours of treatment. A variety of within- and beyond-clinic speech measures were used to assess the clients' posttreatment speech, but James et al. found no evidence that the intensive treatment format produced superior stuttering reductions.

# Speech quality

It has been mentioned previously that prolonged speech treatments may produce speech which sounds and feels unnatural. All clinicians and their potiential clients need to know that. The seriousness of this clinical problem has been noted by Martin, Haroldson and Triden (1984); speech that has an unusual quality is liable to be unacceptable to the client and require excessive levels of attention to maintain. Therefore, the presence of unnatural sounding speech is a likely contributor to the problem of posttreatment relapse. It is interesting to note that this problem is not one that has developed recently. Bormann (1969) cites what appears to be an 18th century description of prolonged speech, and which refers to a trade-off between stutter-free and unnatural-sounding speech. This aspect of the treatment also was noted in Goldiamond's (1965) influential report of the clinical use of prolonged speech.

Regardless of this obvious and long standing problem, little has been done by researchers to offset it. Ingham and Onslow (1987) note that prolonged-speech treatments evolved during an era when there was much concern for the measurement of behaviors that could be directly observed. They suggest that this may have been the reason why measurement of speech naturalness was overlooked. The development of the speech naturalness scale has provided clinicians with a way they can at least attempt to shape natural sounding speech by means of feed-back naturalness scores (see pages 100-101). But evidence from recent years shows that clinicians are still a long way from producing natural sounding-speech in clients they treat with prolonged speech. Table 5 summarizes available data from studies of speech naturalness scores achieved by clients after the transfer portion of their prolonged-speech treatments, and speech naturalness data for control subjects who do not stutter.

The contents of Table 5 are instructive. On any occasion when it is possible to use an RCS-based treatment, that is a desirable option in comparison to prolonged-speech treatment. For perhaps the most problematic aspect of prolonged speech treatments is that, at this stage in their development, it may not be possible to produce natural-sounding speech. This is simply not an issue if the clinician uses RCS treatments to help their clients control stuttering.

TABLE FIVE. Summary results of studies of speech naturalness in controls who do not stutter and clients after the transfer phase of prolonged-speech treatment programs. Values presented are mean scores on a 9-point scale of speech naturalness. Reprinted from Onslow, Hayes, Hutchins and Newman (1992), by permission of the American Speech-Language-Hearing Association.

|  | Runyan, Bell, & Prosek (1990) | Martin, Haroldson, & Triden (1984) | Ingham, Gow, & Costello, (1985) | Onslow, Hayes, Hutchins, & Newman (1992) | Metz, Schiavetti,& Sacco, (1990) |
|---|---|---|---|---|---|
| controls | 2.79 | 2.12 | 2.39 | 3.25 | 3.55 |
| post-transfer clients | - | - | 4.26 | 5.49 | 5.92 |
| difference | - | - | 1.87 | 2.24 | 2.37 |

# Efficiency

As noted before, clients often do not complete intensive prolonged speech programs. This poses a clinical problem, because it is difficult to screen clients to see whether this is likely to happen. The majority of clients can master the speech pattern under intensive conditions, but many cannot use—or choose not to use—that pattern to control stuttered speech during everyday speaking situations. It is only during the transfer phase or the maintenance phase of treatment that the clinician discovers if the technique is ineffective for a client. This can mean that a great deal of the time of the client and clinician is wasted. It is quite likely that all this is a contributing factor to the high rates of posttreatment relapse with intensive prolonged speech treatment; clients may relapse simply because the treatment is unsuitable for them and they should never have been enrolled in the first place. By contrast, RCS treatments permit the clinician to use a set of ABA treatment trials to establish and confirm whether a particular treatment is able to establish and generalize stutter-free speech. An example of this appears in Figure 4 on page 93.

Perhaps the biggest doubt about the efficiency of prolonged speech treatment relates to how clients are instructed. In order for clients to learn the various speech skills involved in prolonged speech, and to retain those skills for a considerable period of time, it is essential to have consistent feedback from clinicians. That is one of the basics of effective teaching. Yet there are serious doubts about whether clinicians can give reliable feedback to clients about target behaviors such as "soft contacts" and "gentle onsets." There is no way to effectively define these target behaviors so that clinicians can be objectively certain about whether a client is or is not using them correctly (Ingham, 1984). They are described in treatment manuals in a vague fashion, with the result that it is mostly not clear to what these labels refer. The term "continuous vocalization," for example, could refer to anything from mumbling to singing. There is an urgent need for clinical research to determine whether clinicians can give consistent feedback to clients about whether they are using prolonged speech correctly. And because intensive prolonged speech treatments normally involve several clinicians, there is a need to determine whether those clinicians agree in the feedback they give to clients in treatment programs. Without such information, clinicians cannot be completely confident about the value of their instruction during prolonged speech treatments.

## Practicality

There are many practical difficulties with prolonged-speech treatments in an intensive format. Such formats are disruptive to normal routines because extraordinary working hours are demanded of clinicians and clients, and other clients' clinic attendances are disrupted while clinicians are fully engaged in operating the program. Nonresidential programs typically operate for at least 12 hours per day and residential programs can require staffing for up to 18 hours per day. With all this in mind a clinician may choose to conduct prolonged speech treatments using the customary once- or twice-weekly visit format. Still, there are practical difficulties associated with this form of treatment. One of those difficulties is that extensive drills in prolonged speech are essential during the treatment and for long periods after the treatment. Yet those drills are tedious and not enjoyable for clients. This problem is especially relevant to the treatment of school-age children. There is no way that the treatment will be successful without such drills, yet only a small portion of children are likely to comply with that treatment requirement.

## Replicability

Replicability of treatments is an essential component of reputable clinical practice. Any clinician who has been adequately trained should be able to conduct any treatment. However, as discussed above, prolonged speech is replicable only in the loosest sense of the word. There is no objective way to determine if a client has achieved "soft contacts," "gentle onsets," "continuous vocalization," and so on. Replicability problems with prolonged speech can mean that clients are restricted to their original treatment facility, because the features of a given prolonged speech treatment cannot be communicated effectively between clinicians. For example, it is difficult to imagine that someone treated with "smooth speech" in Australia who needed assistance in retaining prolonged speech skills could be assisted by a clinician who conducts "precision fluency shaping" in the United States. In contrast, RCS treatments permit clinicians to communicate effectively about the operational features of the treatment. For example, the features of a time-out treatment are simple for any clinician to replicate; the duration of the time-out period, how many stutters occur before a time-out period is imposed, the nature of social and tangible reinforcements, and the extent to which the client imposes time-out in everyday speaking situations.

## Final comments

Numerous doubts have been raised in this and the previous section about the practical and conceptual value of prolonged speech treatments. If these are justifiable queries about this style of treatment, then it remains to be explained why it has been so popular. Shortly after the first Australian investigations were completed on the prolonged speech technique it became obvious that many clinicians considered the procedure to be suitable for all clients. Sixteen years ago, Ingham (1977) commented that there was

> a growing and somewhat alarming trend among many clinicians. This is an apparent inclination to direct subjects to so-called 'intensive treatments'...but clinicians should realize that there is not a shred of evidence which suggests any particular therapy program is likely to be ideal for all individuals. Indeed, it is more likely to be the case that different individuals are suited to different types of therapy procedures. As a matter of course I think every subject should be treated individually within customary clinical conditions. In other words, the clinician's and subject's resources should be used to maximum advantage, before alternate and more demanding types of therapy strategies are introduced. ( pp. 10-11)

One reason that such a situation might have developed was touched on in Wingate's (1971) influential article which suggested that clinicians had a "fear of stuttering." Wingate's paper described clinicians' uncertainties about treating the disorder. Wingate seems to have been correct, because there is convincing survey evidence that clinicians worldwide in the 1980s believed that they were not competent in offering treatment and were ill-informed about stuttering and its treatment (Cooper & Cooper, 1985; Cooper & Rustin, 1985; Lass, Ruscello, Pannbacker, Schmitt, & Everly-Myers; 1989; Mallard, Gardner, & Downey, 1988; St. Louis & Lass, 1981). If clinicians are apprehensive and ill-informed about treatment of stuttering, then this provides a possible explanation for the enormous popularity of pro- longed speech programs in Australia: They offer clinicians a convenient way to circumvent that lack of knowledge by simply referring stuttering clients to intensive treatment centres rather than treating the clients themselves.

If it is the case that intensive treatment facilities are used by clinicians to bypass their lack of treatment knowledge, then there may be a cycle which perpetuates ignorance about appropriate treatment methods. If clinicians are unaware that prolonged speech is a treatment that contains methodological and conceptual shortcomings, they will neither become aware of those shortcomings nor discover alternative treatment approaches without personal experience of prolonged speech in the treatment of stuttering.

# The Role of Support Groups in Prolonged-Speech Treatments[1]

Most countries with well organized treatment services for stuttering also have well organized support groups for those who have the disorder. In Australia, the relevant association is the Australian Speak Easy Association, which consists mostly of people who stutter, but which also maintains links to the speech pathology profession. The Association provides support to those who have had treatment for stuttering and also those who have not had treatment. Its main activities are:

1. Regular meetings among members for the purposes of support and practice of therapeutic techniques. These meetings normally occur in the homes of Association members.
2. Organized activities for people who stutter, such as debating and oratory contests, camps, and programs designed to help maintain the effects of treatment.
3. Provision of public information. The Association has produced several videos, and produces various regular newsletters. Additionally, each year the Association organizes a national "stuttering awareness week."

The Speak Easy Association is obviously an important resource to clinicians. One purpose of clinicians' treatment of stuttering is to assist their clients in the lifelong task of maintaining stutter-free speech. But it is clear that the resources of clinicians are too limited to achieve such a goal without outside assistance. And as mentioned previously, an important part of a stuttering treatment may be to provide various kinds of support to clients, and peer support is an ideal contribution to that treatment goal.

The purpose of this section is to draw attention to some issues that arise from interaction between clinicians and support groups in the treatment of stuttering, and to suggest practical approaches to those issues. In what follows it is suggested that interaction between the speech-pathology profession and the Speak Easy association could rest on recognition of these issues, and also could rest on a clear statement of the contribution that the two groups can make to client management. The Speak Easy Association has contributed much in this regard by making statements of the contribution it can make.[2] Hence much of the following discussion focusses on the contribution that speech pathologists can make to stuttering management.

---

[1] This section is based on Onslow and Costa (1989).

[2] For example, Australian Speak Easy Association (1986) and a distributed pamphlet titled "General Information."

## Professional background

Communication disorders is a diverse field which draws on material from the behavioral and biological sciences (Siegel & Ingham, 1987), and this means that modern clinicians emerge from a broad and comprehensive professional preparation. There is much in this background which equips a clinician with skills to manage stuttering. One example of such skill is modification of human behavior, which qualifies clinicians to help clients control the behavioral disruptions of stuttering. Another skill is understanding of the role of genetics in stuttering, as discusssed in Part Five, which equips clinicians to identify children at risk for developing the disorder.

Misused stuttering treatments can cause considerable harm, and the skills of a professional clinician protect clients from such harm. One example is treatments which involve direct verbal stimulation of children as young as 2 and 3 years, such as that outlined in Part Three. Speak Easy members clearly have become aware of the arrival of such treatments and the rejection of the notion that it is harmful to call attention to early stuttering (Australian Speak Easy Association, 1986). But there is a difference between publicizing new clinical developments and having the skills to implement them with clients. There are critical ethical issues to attend to whenever direct verbal stimulation is applied to a young child (see Part Three). If operant techniques are misused by parents, there could be considerable danger in drawing attention to a child's stuttering. There are many ways that attention can be drawn to stuttering so that a child will suffer significant distress, and there are certainly many parents who are capable of inadvertently causing such a result.

Another example of the value of professional background in stuttering management is treatment choice. There are some clinical decisions to be made about which treatments to use with different clients. It is just not sensible to treat all clients the same way. Yet it appears to be a characteristic of support groups for problem human behaviors that they have a unified advocacy of one particular way of managing problem behaviors. One example is the abstinence approach to problem drinking which Alcoholics Anonymous endorses and around which it constructs its activities. Another example is the approach to problem eating which Weight Watchers endorses during its meetings. The Speak Easy Association shares with these support groups that it builds its regular activities around one particular treatment. That treatment is the prolonged speech technique referred to as "smooth speech":

> The success of the Speak Easy Association revolves around regular maintenance meetings which help members strengthen their fluency skills...Meetings usually start with members speaking at very slow, controlled speeds, then move on through a number of practice areas designed to help members improve their skills. Critiques are given during the evening regarding fluency, content, and present-ation. (Australian Speak Easy Association, 1986).

There are obvious benefits to clients from the publicizing and conduct of such treatment services. However, such activities also could be deleterious in the long-term if they, in effect, encourage the use of one particular treatment strategy for all clients. Stuttering treatments can be based on either prolonged speech or RCS, and can incorporate either programmed or nonprogrammed instruction (see Parts Three and Four). Further, early and advanced stuttering require completely different treatment methods. Input from professional clinicians about the treatment which is suitable for a particular client is a critical part of effective client management.

# Clinical skills

The most valuable contribution of the Speak Easy Association is its assistance with maintenance of treatment benefits: "The main aim of Speak Easy Association in the life of a treated stutterer is to ensure that he or she doesn't slip back into stuttering" (Australian Speak Easy Association, 1986). In order to meet this objective, the Association supplements its regular meetings with a variety of programs and camp-based activities. Of course, this is likely to be of assistance in the maintenance of stutter-free speech. But it is important to recognize several ways that speech pathologists can contribute to the maintenance of stutter-free speech.

There is no doubt that systematic practice of prolonged speech is a contribution to effective maintenance. Every clinician knows that, as do members of the Speak Easy Association:

> It should be noted that, at present, stuttering treatment programmes teach control techniques and do not offer a permanent 'cure' as such. Therefore, a vital aspect following treatment of stuttering, is maintenance. A stutterer, after learning the techniques of controlling his stutter, speaking fluently, and sounding natural, must continue to practice this new found skill in order to maintain fluent speech.[1]

However, maintenance of stutter-free speech depends on the client retaining various prolonged-speech skills (soft contacts, continuous vocalization, and so on) which the clinician taught earlier in the treatment process. Regular practice of those skills is an important part of their retention. However, the emergence of problems in maintaining stutter-free speech may occur because the client begins to lose those clinician-taught skills.[2] In which case, a professional clinician needs to make a contribution to the restoration of those skills so that maintenance can get back on track. Once a client begins to make errors in the basic skills of prolonged speech, continued practice without professional intervention might result in overlearning of errors, which could impede rather than facilitate the maintenance of treatment benefits.

Professional counselling is another clinician skill which makes an indispensible contribution to effective maintenance. Fundamentally, what makes or breaks a prolonged-speech treatment is the skill of the clinician in counselling the client through the difficulties that emerge after stutter-free speech has been instated and generalized. The most successful clinicians in administering prolonged speech treatments are those who have extensive counselling skills, and who can identify the well known signs of impending posttreatment relapse which need to be targeted for counselling. Treatment centres that the author has been associated with have conducted clinics specifically for posttreatment maintenance, and have employed clinicians specifically to direct those clinics.

# Final comments and suggestions

When speech pathologists and the Speak Easy Association work together with stuttering clients, that cooperation needs to occur with full recognition of the role of both parties in maintenance. The Association provides many resources, including support, publicity and speech practice for clients. But there is also a great deal that clinicians can contribute to maintenance. That contribution is not limited to the initial teaching of stutter-free speech. Maintenance is critical in the treatment of advanced stuttering, and clinicians have skills that

---

[1] Pamphlet distributed by the Australian Speak Easy Association; "General Information."

[2] Another possibility—which occurs all too often—is that the skills were not learned correctly in the first place.

are useful during that stage of treatment. If interactions between clinicians and the Association are restricted to the former conducting treatments and the latter conducting maintenance procedures, then the quality of health care for the disorder will suffer.

It is suggested that the issues addressed in this section can be approached in a practical
manner with the adoption of three guidelines to underpin the interaction of clinicians and
support groups in stuttering treatment. First, support groups publicly sanction the treatment
of stuttering, but take steps to avoid direct or implicit endorsement of any particular
treatment procedure. Second, clients are encouraged to consult their original clinician in the
event of posttreatment relapse problems. Finally, for a period of at least one year after
instatement and generalization of treatment gains, the clinician is involved in the conduct of
every client's maintenance. During this period the clinician implements a performance
contingent maintenance program (see Part Two) and provides counselling support for
clients as required. This policy could greatly increase the benefits that clients subsequently
receive from long-term contact with a support group.

# Part Seven:

# Clinical Issues in Management of Early Stuttering

# Diagnosis of Early Stuttering[1]

## Background

The modern trend toward treatment of early stuttering creates a clinical responsibility for early identification. In other words, if clinicians are to treat the disorder as soon as it begins in young children, then they first need to identify when it has begun. However, early identification, in effect, requires a definition of stuttering, and as discussed in Part One, there has been much debate about how to define the disorder but no consensus has been reached. The absence of an accepted definition of stuttering makes it difficult for clinicians to fulfil their responsibility for early identification.

There are several reasons for believing that the development of effective early identification is crucial to the provision of satisfactory clinical services for stuttering. Primarily, it could improve clinicians' capacity to offset the debilitating effects of the disorder in a cost effective manner. Further, it is known that children of people who stutter are particularly susceptible to the disorder (see Part Five). Therefore, effective early identification would enable clinicians to monitor very young children who are known to be genetically at risk of developing stuttering. In this way, any first signs of stuttering in at-risk populations could be managed immediately. Finally, a logical extension of the benefits of early intervention is prevention through screening. Yet screening for the disorder is not possible if clinicians cannot identify it.

In short, there is an urgent need to develop effective strategies for identifying early stuttering. The purpose of this section is to address this need. In so doing, the following suggestions are offered:

1. The problem of identification of early stuttering is one that, for the present, calls for a rational rather than an empirical solution.
2. Identification of early stuttering should provide separately for positive and negative outcomes.
3. All available definitions of stuttering should be harnessed for the purpose of identifying the onset of the disorder.
4. Negative identification should be a conservative process, designed to avoid false negatives.
5. Positive identification should be a comparatively liberal process in relation to negative identification.

## Rational and empirical advances

Empirical research is a useful foundation for clinical practice, so it could be expected to be prominent in the development of strategies to identify early stuttering. Several early

---

[1] This section is based on Onslow (1992a), portions of which are reprinted by permission of the American Speech-Language-Hearing Association.

identification protocols have been suggested (Adams, 1977; Culp, 1984; Curlee, 1980; 1993; Gregory & Hill, 1980; 1993; Johnson, 1980; Pindzola & White, 1986; Riley, 1984; Van Riper, 1971), and these can stimulate many research questions. For example, research might determine the identification accuracy of those protocols, along with their levels of intraobserver and interobserver agreement. In particular, agreement between different clinics in early identification could be established. However, such empirical activity will require many years to complete. For example, the accuracy of identification cannot be determined until the disorder has been unremittingly present for a length of time sufficient to consider it chronic. In most cases, that may take several years.

Desirable as empirical advances are, they are not the only advances that can contribute to progress in the management of communication disorders. Siegel (1987) has argued that, in some cases, progress is possible by rational, rather than by empirical means. Identification of early stuttering is one such case. It would be regrettable if clinicians felt compelled to wait for the output of clinical research before accepting the value of any strategy to identify early stuttering: Their professional responsibilities in that area are too pressing. Accordingly, this section is an attempt to contribute to the work of various authors, mentioned above, in developing clinical protocols for identifying early stuttering. In the interim period until clinical science can adequately address this matter, clinicians need to identify early stuttering using strategies that are logically justifiable. Fortunately, logical advances can be expedient as well as useful.

## Positive identification of early stuttering

Identification of early stuttering amounts in effect to definition of it, and there are several definitions available that might assist clinicians to positively identify early stuttering. These are outlined in Part One. As noted there, a problem with symptomatic definitions is that they are not effective in distinguishing between stutters and normal disfluencies. With very young children, this problem is particularly worrying because of recurring findings that every speech event described in early stuttered speech occurs also in normal speech in the first years of life. These replicated findings seem robust, because they have been derived from direct comparisons of groups of young stuttering and normally speaking children (Bjerkan, 1980; Culp, 1984; Hubbard & Yairi, 1988; Johnson & Associates, 1959; Westby, 1974; Yairi, 1972; Yairi & Lewis, 1984). The Yairi and Lewis (1984) report is particularly impressive among those publications because of the apparent severity of the group of stuttering preschool-age children, who showed a of mean of 21 percent "syllables disfluent" compared to a mean 6 percent "syllables disfluent" in a matched group of normally speaking children. Despite this apparent distinctiveness of the stuttering children, Yairi and Lewis found that, in short (500-syllable) speech samples, every disfluency category that occurred in the speech of stuttering children occurred also in the speech of control children. As indicated in Part One, Perkins' "internal" definition of stuttering also has shortcomings for use with young children. Bloodstein's consensus definition of stuttering also presents no tangible help in identifying early stuttering, because it presents no practical guidelines for reaching a consensus about whether a child's speech is stuttered or normal.

This all represents a problematic state of affairs: Clinicians require a definition to identify cases of early stuttering, but all available definitions have substantial shortcomings. Fortunately, some recent insights of Bloodstein (1990) are useful in addressing such a situation; "we may at different times and for different reasons prefer one or another of these definitions" (p. 392). In other words, judgements about the functional value of definitions should be yoked to the context in which they are used. In day-to-day clinical practice, different definitions of the disorder are applicable to different purposes. For example, a client's self monitoring of stuttered speech beyond the clinic would include internal definition. A within-clinic treatment task might rely on consensus definition, where the combined judgements of clinician and client determine the presence of stuttering. On occasions when clinicians provide information to the public about the disorder, symptomatic definitions might be suitable. This pragmatic approach should be applied to the selection of a definition for use in early identification.

One merit of Bloodstein's consensus definition for positive identification is that it incorporates listener perception. It therefore has content validity because it bypasses difficulties with the limited number of speech events that can be described by symptomatic definitions. Stuttered speech is accompanied by a great number of visual and auditory speech events—some of them extraordinarily subtle—that are not captured by the terms used in symptomatic definitions. A perception-based definition would be able to take account of any and all events that might prompt the perception of stuttered speech.

Another advantage of perception-based identification is its face validity. Early stuttering generally comes to the attention of clinicians because of the perceptions of observers in children's environments. A consensus definition would be able to include the judgements of such observers. Clinicians commonly report the importance of parental concern about stuttering in a diagnostic procedure (for example, Costello, 1983; Starkweather, Gottwald, & Halfond, 1990), and Conture and Caruso (1987) have even gone as far as asserting that the concern of people in a child's environment is essential for a diagnosis of stuttering. In most cases, that concern emerges from parents, whose observations should be considered trustworthy (Riley & Riley, 1983). Curlee (1993) argues that parents are rarely mistaken in believing that their child has begun to stutter. Considering that parents observe their children's speech continuously in a variety of speaking situations, it would be difficult to disregard a parental judgement that a child's speech contained stuttering.

Although a consensus definition of early stuttering is conceptually justifiable, its practical value depends on whether early stuttered speech is readily perceptible. There are a number of sources of support which suggest that this is the case. One such source is grounded in clinical common sense: For the most part, advanced stuttering involves perceptible interruptions in the flow of speech. Therefore the same could be expected of early stuttering. Indirectly, that common sense view is supported by the publications of many researchers. As part of their work, they have allocated subjects younger than 5 years to control and experimental groups by taking account of the perceptions of observers in children's environments and by relating those perceptions to those of clinicians (Adams, 1987; Conture, Rothenberg, & Molitar, 1986; Conture & Kelly, 1991; Hall & Yairi, 1992; Hubbard & Yairi, 1988; Kelly & Conture, 1992; Onslow, Costa, & Rue, 1990; Starkweather & Gottwald, 1993; Yairi & Lewis, 1984; Zebrowski, 1991). In effect, then, these investigators incorporated a consensus procedure in their identification of early stuttering. Parental descriptions of the onset of stuttering (Mowrer, 1987; Rudmin, 1984; Yairi, 1983) certainly support the impression that unusual speech events which are perceptible occur at this time. Of particular note are various parental reports that the onset of stuttering can occur in a single day (see Part One).

As mentioned previously, clinicians have generated many protocols which attempt to carefully specify the features of stuttered speech which can be used to distinguish it from normal speech in the preschool years. This reflects a general belief that the diagnostic task is not straightforward (Bloodstein, 1961). Arguably, the extensive influence of the diagnosogenic theory (see Part Two) may be the origin of that apprehensiveness about diagnosis, because it posited that confusion about stuttered and normal speech actually cause the disorder. Wingate (1988) has argued additionally that the diagnosogenic theory indirectly contributed to that apprehensiveness through research that it prompted. He notes that Johnson's disfluency categories have figured in much of the research which has addressed the issue of differences between early stuttering and normal speech in early childhood. That research has shown an "overlap" between early stuttering and normal speech in preschoolers (see Part One), but this is only to be expected considering that many of Johnson's terms describe normal disfluencies, which could be expected in the speech of both stuttering and nonstuttering preschool children. Hence that research, and many subsequent studies which have replicated its findings (e.g. Bjerkan, 1980; Bloodstein & Grossman, 1981; Conture & Kelly, 1991; Culp, 1984; Hubbard & Yairi, 1988; Yairi, 1972; Yairi & Lewis, 1984; Westby, 1974), could have served to cloud the distinctiveness of early stuttering.

Onslow, Gardner, Bryant, Stuckings and Knight (1992) presented some data pertinent to this matter. From a large collection of recordings of the speech of stuttering and nonstuttering children younger than 5 years, 200 utterances were obtained which contained a single disfluency of some kind. The 200 utterances were presented to clinicians and nonclinicians, who were instructed to indicate whether each disfluency was "stuttering" or "normal." A substantial portion of the utterances were judged with high agreement among listeners to be "stuttering"; 15.5 percent in the case of clinicians and 24.5 percent in the case of nonclinicians. This result was interpreted as an indication that certain speech events are readily perceived as stuttering in young children.

In all, there are grounds for a confident conclusion that early stuttered speech is readily perceptible to observers. Therefore, Bloodstein's consensus procedure could be considered a suitable clinical basis for positive identification of early stuttering. The benefits of such a procedure are its content and face validity, and its congruence with the way that cases of early stuttering are identified by researchers and parents. The perceptually distinctive nature of stuttered speech is *the* most useful identifying feature of the onset of the disorder, and an identification strategy for early stuttering must recognize that distinctiveness.

## Negative identification of early stuttering

There have been many recent attempts to demonstrate the efficacy of early intervention (Coppola & Yairi, 1982; Culp, 1984; Guitar, Schaefer, Donahue-Kilburg, & Bond, 1992; Johnson, 1980; Martin, Kuhl, & Haroldson, 1972; Onslow, Costa, & Rue, 1990; Reed & Godden, 1977; Riley and Riley, 1983; Shine, 1984a; St. Louis, Clausell, Thompson, & Rife, 1982; Stocker & Gerstman, 1983). As this interest in early intervention continues, a corresponding surge should be anticipated in public awareness of the first signs of the disorder and of the availability and value of early intervention services.[1] Predictably, this in turn will result in increased numbers of clinicians seeing children who are suspected of displaying early signs of stuttering. It is likely that many of those children will not have the disorder, leading to an increase in the negative identification rate. In other words, negative identification of early stuttering will become more common as early intervention procedures become more widely known. Additionally, as indicated previously, screening is a logical consequence of recognition of the benefits of early intervention. Because many children who will be screened for stuttering will not have the disorder, screening programs will rely considerably on negative identification procedures.

---

[1] In Australia, treatments for stuttering are regularly featured in media current affairs reports. Additionally, the Australian Speak Easy Association promotes a "National Stuttering Awareness Day," which includes the provision of public information about treatment.

Strategies to identify disorders call for clarification of the relationship between positive and negative identification. For many disorders, negative identification is a direct reciprocal of positive identification. In other words, a person showing no signs of a disorder at one time may be considered to be free of the disorder. However, ascertaining that a young child is free of stuttering is not as straightforward, because stuttering is notorious for its variability across situations (see pages 45-46). In particular, early stuttering typically varies over time, and cases may even present to a clinic without any signs of stuttered speech (see pages 66-67). The variable and episodic nature of early stuttering carries an important implication for negative identification: *A stutter-free speech sample at one point in time is, alone, not a sufficient basis for a decision that a young child is free of the disorder.* Therefore, negative identification is possible only if stuttered speech is absent during the years in which the disorder may begin. In the following section, this long-term view is justified in terms of its capacity to prevent the deleterious effects of false negative identification.

# False positive and false negative identification

Naturally, correct identification is a desirable outcome, whether it involves a child who is stuttering or a child who is not stuttering. However, there are two kinds of errors that may occur. The first of these is a false positive identification, where a nonstuttering child is incorrectly identified as a child who stutters. The second kind of error is false negative identification, where a child who stutters is incorrectly identified as a normally speaking child. Any procedure to identify a disorder carries a false positive identification rate. Faust (1984) has argued that any efficient identification of a disorder should generate few false positive identifications in comparison to true positive identifications. This certainly may be the case with disorders where treatment is either dangerous, lengthy or expensive. However, it is argued below that, in the case of early stuttering, there is little reason for clinicians to be concerned about false positive identification.

Clinicians may be confident that false positive identification will not cause significant harm to a child. Such confidence is buttressed by the increasing rejection in recent years of Johnson's diagnosogenic theory (see Part Five). Further, it is doubtful that a nonstuttering child would be diagnosed as stuttering without good reason. If normal speech perturbations are sufficiently disruptive to a child's speech to suggest that they are stuttering, then treatment might be helpful to that child. It is relevant to note that parents commonly assist children to correct behaviors that are a developmental faltering rather than a pathological condition. For example, parents may assist a 12-month-old child to walk, even though it is not pathological for infants of that age to fall when attempting to walk. Similarly, it should be neither unconscionable, nor unhelpful, to assist a child to overcome speech perturbations that are not part of the condition of stuttering.[1]

In contrast to false positive identification, the prospect of false negative identification of early stuttering is a serious clinical concern. Such errors are potentially harmful to young children, because a lasting and debilitating disorder could develop as a consequence of being overlooked as a target for early intervention. This concern is founded in the common knowledge that treatment of advanced stuttering is much more time consuming, laborious, and prone to failure and relapse, than is treatment of early stuttering. In the case of early stuttering, then, it seems that a modification is needed to Faust's (1984) argument about effective identification. Specifically, it is the number of false negative identifications that

---

[1] Starkweather, Gottwald, & Halfond (1990) describe a case where a child was admitted to their treatment program even though she had what was judged to be normal disfluency.

should be low in comparison to the number of true positive identifications. However, this statement should be considered alongside another perspective of Faust's. This perspective is that the prevalence of a disorder influences the viability of procedures to identify it. In the case of stuttering, one source of information (Andrews, 1984a) indicates that 1.3 percent of 5-year-old children will be stuttering at one time. If this finding is accurate, only 13 children per thousand are targets for positive identification. Taken together, the foregoing considerations have considerable implications for identifying early stuttering: False negative identification rates should be low in relation to a positive identification rate of 13 children per thousand. Even a single false negative identification per thousand children would subject around eight percent of incipient stuttering cases (1 of 13) to a risk of developing a much less tractable version of the disorder later in life.

In summary, it is critical to avoid errors in negative identification of early stuttering, therefore the negative identification process should be as conservative as possible. This conclusion suggests that negative identification might be based on a combination of all three definitions of stuttering discussed previously. In other words, a child's speech should only be identified as nonstuttered if it fails concurrently to conform to symptomatic, internal, and consensus definitions of stuttering. In order to incorporate all definitions, regular observations for the purposes of negative identification could take account of verbal and nonverbal speech events (symptomatic definition), anything that a child verbalizes (e.g. "mummy I can't say it") or parents observe which suggest that a child's speech is affected by a "loss of control" or "involuntary" disruption (internal definition), and whether parents or others in the child's environment have perceived stuttered speech (consensus definition). This strategy, combined with regular observations during the years when stuttering might begin, and the notion that negative identification is not merely a failure to positively identify, provides the most conservative negative identification possible.

# Clinical strategies for identifying early stuttering

The following suggestions about clinical strategies for identification of early stuttering arise from the discussion above:

1. There should be positive and negative components in procedures to identify early stuttering.
2. Positive and negative identification should be nonreciprocal.
3. Some error rate for positive identification is tolerable, therefore positive identifications should be liberal and based on the detection of stuttered speech on one occasion using a consensus definition.
4. The error rate for negative identification should be zero, therefore negative identifications should be extremely conservative and based on repeated observations during the early years of life using all available definitions of stuttering.

The following suggested clinical strategies for identification of early stuttering are based on these conclusions.

## Overview

The strategies involve both a positive and a negative identification component. A child in the positive definition component who is not identified as stuttering is moved to the negative identification component, also referred to as an "at-risk register." This register is a variation of a recommendation by Adams (1977). Such a child remains on the at-risk register for a substantial period of time, until either a clear positive or negative identification occurs. An overview of these strategies is shown in Figure 9.

FIGURE NINE: Diagram of strategies to identify early stuttering, in which positive identification and negative identification are separate and nonreciprocal processes.

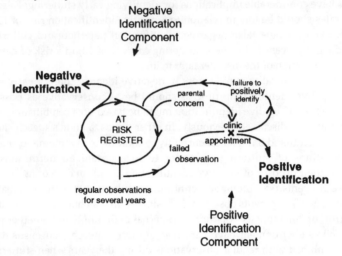

### Positive identification component

In cases of suspected stuttering, the parent/s is given an appointment to bring their child to the clinic along with an audio- or video-tape recording of speech events that are causing concern. Positive identification is based on perception of stuttering in the child's speech either within the clinic or in the audio- or video-tape recording. Positive identification occurs if one parent and a clinician agree on the perception of stuttered speech.

Failures to achieve such consensus about positive identification invoke the following actions. If a parent considers that a child is stuttering, but the clinician fails to perceive stuttered speech in the clinic or in the recording, then the child is placed on an at-risk register. In an instance where a clinician perceives stuttered speech, but a parent does not, positive identification occurs if a second clinician perceives stuttered speech. This judgement by the second clinician may be based on a sample of the client's speech recorded during the clinic visit, and/or on the beyond-clinic audio- or video-tape recording of the child. If the second clinician does not perceive stuttered speech, then the child is placed on an at-risk register.

### At-risk register (negative identification component)

Cases of suspected stuttering who are not positively identified are placed in this component. All children on an at-risk register are observed regularly for a substantial period of time. The clinic could regulate these observations by means of brief parent interviews, or by mail questionnaire. The former option may include telephone calls or face-to-face contact with a clinician or a clinician aide. A more cost effective method for managing an at-risk register might be to instruct parents to telephone the clinic at prescribed intervals. A child's "at-risk" status is not altered if a parent responds negatively to each of the following questions.

Indicate if you have noticed any of the following associated with your child's speech in the past months:

1. Many repetitions of the first part of a word, or a number of words
   (for example "d-d-d-d-daddy" or "I want-want-want-want to play"
   or "can I, can I, can I, can I go to the shop").
2. Periods of silence, or "blocks," when attempting to speak.
3. Prolongation of sounds when attempting to speak (for example,
   "that's a caaaaat").
4. Blinking, facial twitching, or grimacing when attempting to speak.

Indicate if has your child said anything, or you have you noticed anything in the past months that made you think your child has:

5. Had any kind of involuntary disruption of efforts to speak.
6. Lost control of the ability to speak (for example, "mummy I can't
   say it")

Indicate if at any time in the past months,

7. You thought that your child may be stuttering.
8. Someone told you that your child may be stuttering.

It is suggested that these observations occur at 2- or 3-monthly intervals. Children who continue to pass these observations remain on the at-risk register until the clinician is satisfied that a negative identification can be made or until contact with the child is lost. If a child fails an observation because a parent answers "yes" to one of the above questions, that child is routed to the positive identification component and receives a further clinic appointment. A child may also be routed to the positive identification component if a parent becomes concerned about stuttering at any time between observations. A child who is routed to the positive identification component may be positively identified by consensus in the manner described previously. A child who is routed to the positive identification component, but who is not positively identified, is routed back to the at-risk register.

It is difficult to estimate how long a child should remain on the at-risk register before a negative identification can be made. Bloodstein's (1987) review of pertinent literature suggests that the upper limit of such an estimate is 12 years. However, that is likely to be a conservative estimate, which will result in many practical difficulties in maintaining an at-risk register. Perhaps a clinical solution to the problem could incorporate the common belief that the majority of cases of stuttering are likely to begin before the age of 5 years. It may be a justifiable clinical decision to conduct the at-risk register with less frequent observations for older children. For example, 2-year-old children might be observed every 2 or 3 months, but 10-year-old children might be observed every 6 or 12 months.

## Diagnosis and overservicing

The strategies to identify early stuttering suggested in this section raise the issue of overservicing through over-identification. This is because they incorporate the ideas of conservative negative identification and comparitively liberal positive identification. It is a concern that the simultaneous operation of these two factors might effectively pressure clinicians to make positive identifications, with the result that substantial numbers of normal children are erroneously identified as stuttering and receive treatment. However, such a concern would only be justified if positive and negative identification were reciprocal processes. In other words, if the alternative to positive identification was immediate negative identification, it would not be surprising if clinicians overidentified the disorder as a safeguard against false negative identification. However, the strategies outlined in this section place no pressure on clinicians to make positive identifications. Failure to identify stuttered speech on one occasion is not negative identification. Instead, the child is placed on an at-risk register and remains there, if necessary, for several years.

# Choosing a Treatment for Early Stuttering[1]

## Background

The recognition that direct intervention is desirable with early stuttering is a significant development in speech-language pathology, but it is a development that confers on clinicians the responsibility of choosing and justifying a treatment for this group of clients. This responsibility is imposing, because if stuttering is at its most tractable with 2- and 3-year-old children, then management of such cases allows little margin for error in comparison to adult cases. Time wasted with an ill-chosen and ineffective treatment probably will not worsen the condition of an adult client. However, such mismanagement may have significant impact on preschool-age children. At worst, it could result in the development of an intractable and debilitating speech disorder.

At present there are a number of recommended procedures for controlling early stuttering. These procedures are incorporated, either alone or in combination, into treatment programs. This section addresses the advantages, disadvantages, and issues associated with each of these procedures, and presents a position that RCS (operant methodology) is the most justifiable treatment choice for this important group of clients. The discussion takes account of some differences between cases of early and advanced stuttering. These differences should be considered because the unique features of early stuttering may suggest that a unique treatment is required. However, the discussion also takes account of treatments that are known to be useful for adult clients. Finally, considerable value is placed on the results of empirical research pertaining to management of early stuttering.

## Environmental change

As discussed in Part Five, anticipatory struggle theories have in common the idea that stuttering is caused by stressors which relate to speech and communication, and which impact on children during the early stages of speech development. Anticipatory struggle theories suggest that early intervention procedures for stuttering should remove the environmental stressors thought responsible for the development of the disorder. Additionally, the more recent "interactionist" perspective on stuttering suggests that an interaction between physical and environmental influences is responsible for the disorder (see Part Five). That perspective also suggests that manipulating children's environments should be a part of treatment. A survey of the most recently recommended treatments for early stuttering shows that changes to children's speaking environments is the most popular notion about controlling the disorder in early childhood (Ainsworth & Fraser, 1987; ASHA, 1990; Conture, 1982; 1990; Conture & Caruso, 1987; Culp, 1984; Gregory, 1984; 1986; Irwin, 1988; Johnson, 1984; Perkins, 1992; Peters & Guitar, 1990, Prins, 1983; Riley & Riley, 1983; Rustin, 1987; Starkweather, Gottwald, & Halford, 1990; Van Riper, 1973; Wall & Myers,

[1] This section is based on Onslow (1992b), portions of which are reprinted by permission of the American Speech-Language-Hearing Association.

1984; Williams, 1984). Ingham (in press) lists 37 "fluency interruptors" and "fluency facilitators" described in this literature.

## Shortcomings of anticipatory struggle theory

Some of the treatments cited above which involve environmental change are derived from anticipatory struggle explanations of the distal cause of stuttering. This provides a starting place for evaluating their merit. Indeed, the value of such a treatment is limited intrinsically by the value of its supporting theory. Therefore, in addressing the merits of environmental change as an early intervention for stuttering, first consideration is given to the merits of anticipatory struggle theory. As discussed in Part Five, there are good reasons to question the credibility of anticipatory struggle theory. From a scholarly viewpoint, those reservations do not close the matter, because all theories to date about the cause of stuttering have encountered serious difficulties. However, from a clinical perspective, a conclusion about the value of anticipatory struggle theory is a different matter, because it will have consequences for the health care of clients. Clinical practice involves day-to-day provision of accountable, documented and conceptually justifiable health care services to those who seek help with stuttering. Because anticipatory struggle theories have not been directly tested, and because they have shortcomings in explanatory power, they may be questionable bases for the provision of such care.

## Lack of empirical evidence for environmental change treatments

There is a general lack of empirical support for treatment programs which modify the environment of children who begin to stutter (Costello, 1983; Ingham, 1993). Some studies pertinent to the issue exist, and have not provided encouraging results. Cox, Seider & Kidd (1984) searched fruitlessly for environmental factors that might separate families without stuttering members from families with many stuttering members (see Part Five). Meyers and Freeman (1985a) found that mothers of stuttering children did not characteristically interrupt the speech of their children when compared to mothers of nonstuttering children. However, they found that mothers of stuttering and nonstuttering children were more likely to interrrupt a child during a disfluency than during passages of speech without disfluency. Ratner (1992) showed that reduction of parental rate and complexity of speech did not influence any speech behaviors of preschool-age children. Another negative result was presented by Weiss and Zebrowski (1992). Anticipatory struggle theory predicts that children will be more disfluent when responding to questions from their parents than when they are making assertions. However, Weiss and Zebrowski found that nonstuttering children were more disfluent when making assertions. Starkweather and Gottwald (1993) found low but nonsignificant correlations between stuttering severity and variables of parental speech rate and number of parental interruptions.

Some reports have suggested that there is a relation between parents' speech rate and stuttering rate in children (Guitar, Schaefer, Donahue-Kilburg, & Bond, 1992; Meyers & Freeman, 1985b; Stephenson-Opsal & Bernstein-Ratner, 1988). A study by Kelly and Conture (1992) explored speech rates, interrupting behaviors, and response time latencies during conversation for two groups of parent-child dyads. One group contained children who stuttered and the other contained nonstuttering children. No significant differences were found between groups of children or parents that were consistent with the presence of environmental stressors related to stuttering. Kelly and Conture did report a correlation between the children's stuttering severity and the extent to which their parents spoke at the same time as their children.

The overall meaning of the studies described above is difficult to interpret because of their mixed results. The results are certainly too premature for a conclusion that stressors in children's environments can be changed to control their stuttering. If such stressors played a role in stuttering treatment, then it would be expected that researchers could measure such effects and replicate their findings on many occasions. It is clear that much work remains to be done if convincing empirical support for anticipatory struggle theory is to be generated. In particular, it is troubling that environmental change treatments have attracted virtually no direct clinical trials based on beyond-clinic speech data and sound treatment evaluation principles. During a clinical era lasting many decades—from the time of the diagnosogenic theory—when these procedures have been the most favored ones for early intervention, there has been only one very preliminary clinical trial of those procedures (Guitar, Schaefer, Donahue-Kilburg, & Bond, 1992), which provided indecisive results.[1]

# Variants of prolonged speech

Treatment modelled on prolonged speech has dominated management of advanced stuttering for the past two decades, with many existing variations of prolonged speech. These treatments have been shown to be of value with adults in extensive clinical trials over two decades. As discussed in Part Six, the extent to which prolonged speech treatments are effective is a matter for some debate, but there is no doubt that they can assist some clients to eliminate most of their stuttering for a significant period of time.

Considering the extensive popularity of prolonged speech treatments, it is not surprising that variants of them have been adapted for use with very young children. As noted in Part Six, many preschool clients of Australian clinicians reportedly were treated with procedures based on prolonged speech. This finding is reflected in recent clinical writings. There are numerous recommendations for how the procedure should be adapted to manage cases of early stuttering. For example, Johnson (1984) prescribes that "effortless, smooth, continuous breath flow" and reduced speech rate should be taught with parental modelling, and Culp (1984) refers to "easy speech" which "is an exaggerated, soft, slow…speech pattern in which vowels are slightly prolonged and normal stress, intonation and juncture are maintained" (p. 42). Gregory (1986) also refers to "easy speech," described in this instance as "a slightly slower than normal rate with easy initiations and smooth transitions" (p. 33). Conture (1990) recommends a variety of analogies for use when teaching a prolonged speech to children, and Shine (1984b) describes programmed instruction in an "easy-speaking voice" that incorporates "easy onset" and "continuous airflow." Starkweather, Gottwald, and Halfond (1990) also incorporate such techniques in their treatment program, as do Peters and Guitar (1991). Runyan and Runyan (1993) report the use of their treatment program with preschool children, in which they adapt prolonged speech terminology and instruction; for example, "turtle speech" (p. 102) for reduced speech rate, "start Mr voice box running smoothly" (p. 106) for gentle onsets and "touch the 'speech helpers' together lightly" (p. 107) for soft contacts.

---

[1] There have been many anecdotal reports of the success of environmental change treatments. For example, Starkweather, Gottwald, and Halfond (1990) reported that, over a 9-year period, 29 stuttering children have completed their treatment program which is based on the demands and capacities model (see page 138). They report that all those children stopped stuttering. Williams (1984) reported that "approximately 90 percent of the children I see…regain normal fluency. (p. 26). However, neither a treatment evaluation design nor speech data are presented in support of such claims.

## Advantages and disadvantages of prolonged speech as an early intervention

*Theoretical soundness*

Variants of prolonged speech might be considered a suitable treatment for early stuttering for the same reason that they are considered a suitable treatment for advanced stuttering. Namely, there is abundant evidence that stuttering involves speech motor dysfunction (see Part Five), and speech pattern changes obviously involve an alteration to speech motor processes. Some important evidence for abnormal speech motor functioning has been found at the level of acoustic analysis, in the sense that the acoustic signal reflects speech motor activity. The stutter-free speech of adults who stutter has been shown, with few exceptions (Watson & Alfonso, 1982; Zebrowski, Conture, & Cudahy, 1985) to contain longer acoustic segment durations than found in nonstuttering speakers (Borden, Baer, & Kenney, 1985; Borden, Kim & Spiegler, 1987; Di Simoni, 1974; Healey & Gutkin, 1984; Healey & Ramig, 1986; Hillman & Gilbert, 1977; Horii & Ramig, 1987; Love & Jeffress, 1971; Metz, Conture & Caruso, 1979; Pindzola, 1987; Shenker & Finn, 1985; Starkweather & Myers, 1979). Further, it is well known that one effect of treatments based on prolonged speech is to promote lengthening of such segment durations (Metz, Onufrack, & Ogburn, 1979; Mallard & Westbrook, 1985; Metz, Samar & Sacco, 1983; Ramig, 1984; Webster, Morgan, & Cannon, 1987). One interpretation of these effects is that such acoustic variables have a functional relationship to stuttering frequency (Onslow & Ingham, 1987). Accordingly, the extended durations of acoustic segments found in stuttered speech might reflect the speaker's attempts to overcome their speech motor deficit, and the extension of such segments during treatments based on prolonged speech could further assist in controlling the motor deficits involved with the disorder (Onslow, van Doorn, & Newman, 1992).

It should not be too difficult to go one step further and suggest that, in addition to adults, recovery from stuttering in young children might occur through speech motor alterations. Such a thought is justified by findings that the unusually long acoustic durations in the stutter-free speech of adult stutterers is present also in children who stutter (Adams, 1987; Robb, Lybolt & Price, 1985; Winkler & Ramig, 1986). Indeed, it is conceivable that, independent of the efforts of clinicians, speech motor adjustment plays an important part in recovery from early stuttering. It certainly is the case that such motor adjustments might explain much of what is known about early stuttering. For example, its well-known tractability might be interpreted as a reflection of the capacity of preschool children to make the necessary speech motor change to control their disorder, before speech motor behavior becomes immutable with increasing age. Additionally, the phenomenon of "spontaneous recovery" from early stuttering might be interpreted in part as a maturational effect that produces changes in children's speech motor systems.

*Lack of empirical support*

It would be incautious to assume that preschool-age children who stutter will respond to treatments based on prolonged speech in the same way that adults respond. Therefore, clinicians need reports of the effectiveness of this procedure with cases of early stuttering to assist them in deciding whether it is an acceptable treatment for that age group.

Unfortunately, available information about the effect of prolonged speech instruction on the stuttering of preschool-age children is of a preliminary nature and quite unconvincing. Shine (1984a) presented, for 14 children, "pretest," "post- test," and "follow-up" data which showed greatly reduced stuttering following treatment. It is not clear from the report how many of these children were of preschool age, however their age range was 2 years 9 months to 8 years 0 months, with a mean age of 4.9 years. Shine's report stated only that follow-up data were collected at variable periods from 1 to 5 years. No information was provided about the duration or nature of assessment speech samples, nor where the samples were collected. Data were presented in measures of "stuttered words per minute," which is a virtually impossible measure to interpret because little is known about the speech rates of preschool children, and also because reliability assessment did not accompany the data. Culp (1984) presented data on 14 children at the completion of a treatment program which showed reduced stuttering in five, 150-syllable clinic speaking situations. These data are difficult to interpret because the constituents of Culp's "percent disfluency" measure were not specified.[1] It is also not possible to know the extent to which Culp's data described the effect of procedures based on prolonged speech, because the program incorporated environmental change strategies. Recurring shortcomings in the above reports are the unevaluated reliability of their data and the absence of evidence for generalization of treatment effects beyond the clinic. As such, it is not possible to interpret them as indicators of the effectiveness of this treatment for preschool-age children.

### Practical difficulties

There are numerous problems intrinsic to prolonged speech treatment. These problems were discussed in detail in Part Six, but the problem of practicality is particularly relevant to their use with young children. With older clients, establishing stutter-free prolonged speech is quite an arduous and intrinsically unappealing process. Considering the limited perseverance and task orientation of very young children, such procedures might be regarded as dubious for use with such clients. Nonetheless, proponents of variants of prolonged speech for early stuttering do not make it clear how prolonged speech should be established in young children. Nor is it clear how generalization should be achieved. Once the stutter-free prolonged speech is learned, adult clients then purposefully attempt to use this pattern in everyday speech situations. How preschool-age children might be prevailed on to use prolonged speech in everyday speaking situations is unclear. At the very least, successful establishment and generalization of prolonged speech in 2- and 3-year-old children is a process that would involve much repetitive speech training and drilling, but such a process is unlikely to be able to be made appealing to young children. It would be equally unappealing for young clients if prolonged speech sounded unusual, yet such treatments are notorious for producing unusual-sounding speech as well as stutter-free speech in adult clients (see Part Six). If it is unlikely that adults will show long-term compliance in using an unusual speech pattern (Martin, Haroldson, & Triden, 1984), then it is even less likely that a preschool-age child would persist with such a pattern.

There is one potentially serious consequence of the practical difficulties with prolonged speech procedures applied to early stuttering: Their successful execution is dependent on the age of the child. The ultimate purpose of the development of early intervention should be to establish procedures to eliminate the first signs of stuttering. But it is clear that children as young as 2 years would not comply with prolonged speech procedures, and, consequently, this would delay treatment. For this reason, any trend for clinicians to treat preschool-age children with versions of prolonged speech could undermine the development of optimal early intervention services for this disorder.

---

[1] For example, it is not clear whether "disfluency" includes only stutterings, or normal disfluencies as well. It also is not clear whether "percentage" refers to syllables, words, utterances, or sentences.

*Conceptual difficulties*

In Part Two it was argued that it is unwise to assume that a client has insufficient skill to produce stutter-free speech. Yet it is often overlooked that prolonged speech treatments operate with exactly that assumption. Treatments based on prolonged speech provide clients with those skills that they do not have by replacing stuttered speech with prolonged speech. In the case of adult clients, the assumption that their problem amounts to a skill deficit may be warranted. The notorious intractability of stuttering throughout the adult years of life certainly suggests as much. However, with the early stages of the disorder, such an assumption may not be as justifiable. As Bellack and Hersen (1977) have pointed out (see Part Two), problem behaviors, particularly those of children, do not necessarily imply a skill deficit. Indeed, there are excellent reasons to believe that early stuttering may be an instance of the problem behaviors referred to by Bellack and Hersen which do not involve a skill deficit. In other words, stutter-free speech is probably more within the behavioral capabilities of preschool-age children than is the case with adults. Hence it would be difficult to justify the selection of a variant of prolonged speech as a first treatment of choice.

# Response contingent stimulation (operant methodology)

Another treatment for early stuttering is that which incorporates response contingent stimulation (RCS), or operant methodology. The previous suggestion that early stuttering may not represent a skill deficit implies that operant methods may be helpful in its management, as they are for many problem behaviors of early childhood. The following sections consider the advantages and the disadvantages of RCS procedures as the bases for early intervention for stuttering.

## Advantages of RCS as an early intervention

*Indirect and direct empirical support*

As outlined in Part Five, operant methodology is known to have controlling effects with adults who stutter. Studies with a variety of verbal and nonverbal stimuli permit a conclusion that stuttering mostly can be ameliorated by such stimuli in laboratory settings, and that this effect is clinically useful. Also there are data which suggest that operant methodology with children beyond preschool age can be the basis of an effective treatment. Such information about the effects of RCS on stuttering provides some indirect support for the use of such procedures with very young children. That indirect empirical support is enhanced by recent reappraisals of literature dealing with so-called "spontaneous recovery" from stuttering. As discussed in Part One, those reappraisals have provided credible suggestions that verbal stimulation from the environments of incipient stuttering children— much of it likely to be contingent—contributes to clinic-free recovery from the disorder in the early years of life. This is of particular interest because it suggests that parents of incipient stuttering children might be able to conduct informally managed interventions for the disorder that are based on operant methodology.

Some limited outcome data are available for early interventions based on RCS. The Martin, Kuhl, and Haroldson (1972) and Reed and Godden (1977) reports (see part Five) included data for preschool-age subjects for posttreatment periods ranging from 8 to 13 months. For those subjects, stuttering reductions were durable for those periods. Onslow, Costa & Rue (1990) constructed a treatment program based on verbal RCS. This program was administered by parents in the everyday speaking environments of incipient stuttering children. A case study of this treatment was reported for four children younger than 5 years. The speech of the children was assessed repeatedly over a 2-month pretreatment period and over a 9-month posttreatment period. A 9-month posttreatment assessment showed that, in all within- and beyond-clinic speaking situations, the stuttering of the children had reduced to a range of 0-2 %SS. This result was comparable, or superior to, the results reported for adult treatments based on prolonged speech.

To use the above evidence in support of RCS is only to cite a slight advantage over other contenders for early intervention. The evidence concerned amounts only to three studies involving a handful of children. Further, as discussed in Part Five, the Martin, Kuhl, and Haroldson (1972) and Reed and Godden (1977) studies contain serious shortcomings. Also, the Onslow, Costa and Rue (1990) report cannot be considered a tight demonstration of the beneficial effects on RCS on early stuttering. Nonetheless, those studies are interpretable because each demonstrated the reliability of their stutter-count measures, and each demonstrated that their effects generalized to beyond-clinic speaking situations.

*Simplicity*

One compelling advantage of operant methodology as an intervention for early stuttering is that it is simpler than those that require an alteration either to the child's environment or to the client's speech pattern. As discussed previously, it would be an elaborate matter to modify environmental stressors which include parental attitudes, expectations and behavior, and to teach prolonged speech to preschool-age children.

The simplicity of RCS treatments could be beneficial in treatment of early stuttering in several ways. First, RCS procedures might be expected to be more time efficient than procedures to restructure clients' living environments or their customary way of speaking; the reports of Martin, Kuhl and Haroldson (1972) and Reed and Godden (1977) showed clinically significant effects in a matter of several hours.

The simplicity of RCS-based treatments also means that the clinical skills required for their conduct are commonplace. The basics of RCS are not specialized skills, and can be administered by any properly trained clinician. Because of this, a goal of effective early intervention is more likely to be achieved because all clinicians are able to contribute to it. But more importantly, the basic principles of operant methodology should be able to be mastered by most parents, facilitating a further improvement in the cost effectiveness of treatment. In fact, as noted in Part Two, systematic RCS can be thought of as merely an extension and formalization of many parenting skills that are brought to bear on a number of problem behaviors of early childhood. And the well known effectiveness of RCS with children might be partially attributed to the fact that parents have access to reinforcers that are potent for children.

A final benefit of the simplicity of RCS procedures is that they are replicable because their components can be documented in objective terms (Onslow & Ingham, 1989). This is a sharp contrast to the poorly specified dimensions of environmental change discussed previously, and a contrast also to the nature of speech patterns currently used in treatment, which defy operationalization (see Part Six). Onslow and Ingham (1989) have argued that the replicability of RCS is of benefit to the clinical community because precise knowledge about the nature of treatments can be shared. But a more important foreseeable benefit to clinicians is that the replicable operations of RCS might encourage far more treatment outcome research than the poorly specified procedures of environmental change and prolonged speech variants.

## Disadvantages of RCS as an early intervention

*Failure to replicate previous studies*

It would not be surprising if clinicians were apprehensive about the lack of systematic replication of the laboratory findings about the controlling effects of RCS on early stuttering (Martin, Kuhl & Haroldson, 1972; Reed & Godden, 1977). Indeed, considering their characteristic replicability, it is reasonable to expect that those findings would be systematically replicated. Yet this has been far from the case. More than 20 years have elapsed since publication of the Martin et al. data, and no replication has occurred. The Reed and Godden article cannot be accepted as a replication of the puppet study, because it used a different stimulus, it failed to show the controlling effects of that stimulus, and it was restricted to one subject in the same age group. The results of Onslow, Costa, & Rue (1990) also contribute little in the way of replication because, as indicated previously, those results were not an experimental demonstration of the effects of RCS. In short, the beneficial effects of the TO procedure on early stuttering were potentially the most important empirical finding about the disorder in recent decades, but that potential has not been realized experimentally.

This state of affairs presents a caveat to any confidence placed in operant methodology as an early intervention, and invites speculation about failure to replicate. Certainly, the original TO findings were of sufficient interest to generate research. In fact, they could not have been regarded as anything but startling. Ingham (1984) touched on one possible explanation; the influence of the diagnosogenic theory prompted their oversight by researchers and clinicians. Another explanation is that the results of the original RCS studies were in fact not overlooked, and that numerous attempts at replication occurred but failed. In the case of single-subject designs, such as those used by Martin et al., positive results may be favored over negative results for publication, because firm interpretation is possible only when positive results occur. Conceivably, then, the original promise of the Martin et al. (1972) and the Reed and Godden (1977) reports was pursued but not substantiated, unbeknown to the scientific community.

# Conclusions and final comments

One purpose of this section was to discuss advantages and disadvantages of different procedures for early intervention with stuttering. A conclusion to emerge from these discussions is that there is little reason for clinicians to be satisfied with *any* kind of treatment they can provide for children who begin to stutter. All available treatments show deficits in one or more of the areas of conceptualization, specificity, and empirical verification. Considering speech pathologists' critical need for justifiable early intervention procedures for stuttering, this is an alarming situation.

Another conclusion to this section is that there are some reservations about treatments that are based on manipulating children's environments. The line of theoretical reasoning about the cause of stuttering, which underpins those treatments, stretches credulity somewhat because of shortcomings in its explanatory power and its lack of empirical verification. Further, after many decades of popularity, the clinical practice of environmental change has not been verified empirically. Considering the imposition that such practices make on families' lifestyles, this is a surprising deficit in a profession that has distinguished itself by its concern for accountability. It is little wonder that the ethics of such treatment practices has been challenged (Costello, 1983; Ingham, in press). It is particularly questionable that a clinician might, with dataless treatment practices, imply that a home environment causes or perpetuates stuttering in a young child. Continuing endorsement of environmental change procedures can only be conditional on the appearance of supportive data.

The value of variants of prolonged speech in early intervention could be argued from the perspective of stuttering as a problem of speech motor control. From this viewpoint, there is some justification for using prolonged speech to help very young children to control stuttered speech. But without procedural details about how this might be accomplished, and without the results of sound clinical trials, it is impossible to recommend that such techniques are a part of early intervention procedures. Recommendations to use prolonged speech with early stuttering probably reflect the historical popularity of this style of treatment rather than its suitability for the age group concerned.

There could be detrimental consequences if preschool children are encouraged to speak with an unusual speech pattern. Such procedures could prove to be as beneficial for young children as they are for adults. But little is known about early neuromotor speech development, and the effects of such speech pattern changes on 2- and 3-year-old children are unpredictable. Conceivably, such changes could impact substantively and unpredictably on a developing speech neuromotor system (A. Packman, personal communication, 1992). It is also possible that the development of early intervention procedures may be hindered if variants of prolonged speech achieve widespread popularity for treatment of early stuttering, because the successful utilization of those procedures is age dependent.

The most positive conclusion resulting from this section relates to the potential of RCS as an early intervention technique. In spite of several shortcomings, such procedures are particularly suitable for use with young children, they are known empirically to control stuttering in older adults and older children, and clinicians should be able to use them efficiently and without additional training because of their simplicity. Finally, there is direct scientific evidence that demonstrates their potential. Other early intervention procedures considered in this section share few of these advantages. Although a conclusion about the merits of RCS may be positive, it should also be a carefully guarded one. Some initial, startling laboratory findings about the effectiveness of those procedures have not been replicated even once over a period of nearly 20 years. Further, there are only preliminary data to describe the effectiveness of operant methodology as a basis for early intervention programs. Obviously, continued research efforts will be required to convince clinicians of the merit of such procedures.

One development considered in this section has been the arrival of the "interactionist" (Conture & Caruso, 1987) model for the treatment of early stuttering; the view that stuttering results from an interaction between a child's capacities for "fluent speech" and the environment. As suggested in Part Five, this development retains the relevance of environmental influences in stuttering, largely in the form they were described in anticipatory struggle theory, but combines them with an acknowledgment of the role of factors intrinsic to the child. Such a treatment model may have some negative features. First, it is almost completely non-directive, providing neither theoretical nor practical direction for clinicians. Virtually any clinical practice could be justified from within such a framework (A. Packman, personal communication, 1993). Any aspect of a child's motor, emotional, cognitive or linguistic development could be altered in the interests of promoting "capacity for fluent speech," and virtually any aspect of a child's environment could be modified on suspicion that it might be precipitating or maintaining stuttered speech. This situation is not conducive to the development of early intervention for stuttering. For example, the "interactionist" model has led some clinicians to combine two of the treatment categories described in this section into the one treatment; manipulating aspects of a child's environment and at the same time using variants of prolonged speech to enhance "capacity for fluent speech" (for example, Gregory, 1986; Johnson, 1984; Starkweather, Gottwald, & Halfond, 1990; Culp, 1984). From the viewpoint of service provision that may not be a bad thing, but it is not desirable from the viewpoint of discovering the identity of effective treatment agents for children who begin to stutter. For example, Starkweather et al. report good results from their treatment which involves environmental change according to the demands and capacities model (see footnote, page 181). But in that program the clinicians may also teach the child to

> "produce speech at a slow rate...accomplished by stretching all continuant sounds. Connect words within phrases to reduce choppiness...fluency-shaping techniques such as gentle or easy onset, light articulatory contacts, and good resonance. Frequently, a combination of these approaches is necessary to bring about the most rapid change." (p. 99)

Interactions of the treatment methods considered in this section may occur even without the intention of clinicians. For example, the RCS-based treatment described in Part Three may inadvertently change children's environments in many of the ways that clinicians purposefully do in other treatments. This might occur because parental RCS needs to be conducted in an atmosphere of support and positiveness. Such an atmosphere may serve to eliminate many of the pressures speculated to be involved with stuttering. Another example would be where a child is encouraged to use "soft contacts," "gentle onsets," or any other of the components of prolonged speech. It is quite conceivable that parents, in effect, might provide RCS for stuttering if they encourage their child to repeat stuttered utterances with those features of prolonged speech. It is also conceivable that attempts to produce less stressful speaking environments for children might promote an alteration to customary speech; especially if the parents reduce their speech rate and encourage a "relaxed" style of communicating with their children.

Even more likely is that RCS treatments for stuttering promote changes to customary speech patterns (Prins & Hubbard, 1988). This might explain why very young children recover from the disorder with striking ease compared to adults; young children can easily adjust their speech motor functioning because they have not completed their neurological development. A preliminary report by Packman, van Doorn, and Onslow (1992) presented acoustic analyses of the speech of two preschool-age children who received the treatment described in Part Two. Data showed posttreatment acoustic changes in these children which were similar to those reported for older children and adults who had been treated with prolonged speech (Onslow, van Doorn, & Newman, 1992; Packman, Onslow, & van Doorn, in press). Replication of these findings may present an avenue for research into the mechanisms by which RCS controls early stuttering.[1]

In short, there is a critical need for information about the potential for variables considered in this section to control stuttering; environmental change, prolonged speech and RCS. Without that information it is difficult to foresee any powerful developments in treatments for early stuttering. Even a large body of anecdotal evidence and extensive clinical trialing of early intervention programs will not contribute much to teasing out the role of variables in controlling early stuttering and how those variables may interact. That block to clinical research is perhaps the most concerning feature of early intervention

---

[1] If the effects of RCS on early stuttering occur because children make some kind of change to the way that they speak, then this would raise another objection to the use of prolonged speech as a treatment for such children; teaching an unusual speech pattern to a child may discourage the child from using self-generated controls over stuttering (A. Packman, personal communication, 1993).

practices considered in this section. The only way to overcome that block may be to look to the research laboratory for information about the control of early stuttering through the experimental analysis of behavior (see page 118). The benefits of such research have been demonstrated already with RCS (Martin, Kuhl, & Haroldson, 1972; Reed & Godden, 1977), and clinicians sorely need such information about the role of environmental change and prolonged speech as variables that can control early stuttering.

# The Value of
# Early Intervention

## The issue

There is no doubt that a portion of children who begin to stutter recover without formally conducted treatment and without regular attendance with their parents at a speech clinic. This raises an important issue concerning service provision for early stuttering. Starkweather (1990) has noted that modern treatment programs for early stuttering have in common the philosophy that it is better to treat children "whose speech shows evidence of abnormal disfluency" (p. 82), rather than wait to see if recovery will occur. Riley and Riley (1983) agree:

> Every child who exhibits abnormal disfluencies should be seen within a few months of stuttering onset....Such early intervention introduces the possibility that some children whose stuttering seems chronic, but who will outgrow their stuttering anyway, will be treated during their preschool years. This is not a very strong argument against early intervention, given the social benefits of an early remediation of stuttering as weighted against the possibility of much more complex, lengthy, and costly treatment later on. (p. 44)

However, as Starkweather has noted elsewhere (Starkweather & Gottwald, 1993), the matter is far from closed. Martin and Lindamood (1986) comment that the actual portion of cases of early stuttering which recover without formal treatment will influence the health care services which need to be directed to early stuttering. Andrews (1984a) has argued that early intervention for stuttering is an inefficient use of health care resources because it will waste those resources on children who will recover. Hence, Andrews suggests that clinicians direct treatment services to children whose stuttering persists:

> if the majority of preschool stutterers is likely to recover within a year, then treatment of most very young stutterers is not likely to be cost effective, and speech-language pathologists should give first priority to treating children whose stutter is persisting. ( p. 11)

and

> if parents of young stutterers are concerned about their children's speech they should be counseled about coping with the child's difficulties and reminded that 60% of children who have stuttered for less than 1 year can be expected to recover without active treatment (p. 11).

This view opposes the notion that treatment should begin at the first signs of stuttering, and introduces the idea that a delay of some duration is appropriate before intervention. Curlee (1993) shares this view:

> while most children who begin to stutter do not require direct clinical management, they should be monitored systematically for at least a year after onset. Monitoring only, or accompanied by indirect treatment procedures, should continue until there is no improvement or there is remission of stuttering. Direct treatment should begin once a child evidences persistent signs of chronic stuttering. (p. 20)

Yairi, Ambrose, and Niermann (1993) are more cautious:

> Our cumulative longitudinal findings seem to raise questions about the advisability of advocating immediate intervention...especially in cases of early

referrals. Alternative strategies, such as a waiting period, immediate direct intervention, or indirect intervention, should be the focus of careful research. (p. 527)

Clinicians need to make a decision about this matter, and some pertinent considerations in making that decision are discussed below.

# Does early stuttering distress children?

Stuttering is obviously a disorder that can cause distress to adults, so this raises a suspicion that it might distress young children. If, on the whole, the onset of stuttering does not cause significant distress to young children, then this might support the suggestion that treatment could be withheld for a period. Some early conceptualizations of the onset of stuttering, such as those by Bluemel and Johnson (see Part Five), held that children were unconcerned by their speech at the first signs of stuttering. Bloodstein (1987) and Van Riper (1982) support this view to the extent that they believe that any chronic distress occurs late in the course of the disorder. However, in their summaries of their clinical observations, both these writers mention that children may show some concern at the signs of early stuttering. In particular, Bloodstein indicates that

> it is commonplace for children as young as two or three to show acute frustration when they stutter by refusing to speak, crying, beating the wall with their hands, or saying, "Why can't I talk?" (Bloodstein, 1987, p. 42)

This appears to be common knowledge among clinicians. A recently published anecdotal example is Ingham's (1993) remarks that "frustration, anger, or bewilderment" (p. 69) in a child are among the diagnostic signs of stuttering.

There are some empirical reports which describe children's reactions during the early stages of stuttering. Johnson and Associates (1959) interviewed parents with extensive questionnares. In Study III, 150 sets of parents were interviewed, and the findings presented below are from that study with the exception of two pieces of data from Study II, which was based on 50 sets of parents. Johnson and Associates asked questions of mothers and fathers separately, but only the mothers' responses are mentioned below.[1] Yairi (1983) interviewed 22 parents with a questionnaire, and Onslow, Harrison, and Jones (1993) received through the mail 121 questionnaires which had been completed by parents of stuttering preschool children.

Yairi reported that 22.7 percent of parents said their child was aware of stuttering when it first began, and Onslow et. al reported a figure 37.0 percent. Yairi reported that 18.2 percent of parents said their child was "bothered" by stuttering when it first began. Figures pertaining to this matter presented by Johnson and Associates are much lower. Only 11.3 percent of parents reported that the child was aware of stuttering when it first began, and only 5.1 percent reportedly showed "surprise" or "bewilderment." And only 12.8 percent of Johnson and Associates' surveyed parents thought that early stuttering was "unpleasant" for their child, and only 11.5 percent of them thought that the child was "irritated" by it.

Johnson et al. reported that 17.5 percent of parents stated that their child avoided speaking situations at some time after the start of stuttering, and Onslow et. al reported a figure of 20.5 percent. Johnson et al. asked parents how sensitive their child was about stuttering (Study II), and 78.0 percent said that their child was either "very," "moderately," or

---

[1] There are some difficulties in interpreting Johnson and Associates' data. Their stuttering subjects were recruited on the basis of parental belief that the child was stuttering. However, they report that, in Study III, 47 of the 150 experimental children were not considered to be stuttering by the interviewers at the time of interview.

"mildly" sensitive. The remaining 22.0 percent of parents said that the child was not sensitive and not did not "feel there is anything wrong with his speech." They also asked parents how their children reacted to their stuttering, and 23.3 percent in Study II and 14.2 percent in Study III responded that the child either appeared "disgusted," "embarrassed," "angry," "irritated," "frustrated," or stamped their foot or said "I can't say it." In the Onslow et al. study, 30.8 percent of parents reported that their child said something to indicate being distressed by stuttering during an average period of around one year post onset. The parents were asked to write down why they believed their child was distressed, and some surprisingly extreme responses were reported. For example,

> She would put her hand to her mouth, and she would get angry with herself and sometimes hit her mouth with her hand and say 'I can't say it.'

> He was asking for a drink and got stuck on the words 'can', 'I', 'a' and before finishing slumped to the floor, cried and said he couldn't talk any more.

> He kept hitting his mouth as if his mouth was being naughty and required a smack and this was pathetic to watch. Two relatives were in tears when they saw this frustration he had when trying to speak.

> He gave up talking and resorted to pointing to objects and only saying 'that.'

Some data pertinent to this matter were reported recently by De Nil and Brutten (1991). Adults who stutter are thought to have negative attitudes to speaking compared to other speakers. That is not surprising, but DeNil and Brutten used a measure of attitude to speech to show that the same thing might pertain to children. The measure used was a survey which required 63 children who stuttered to answer "true" or "false" to 32 questions such as "it is hard for me to talk to strangers," "people worry about the way I talk," and "my words don't come out easily." Results showed that stuttering children as young as 7 years scored much differently on the measure of attitude to speech than did nonstuttering 7-year olds. As considered in a later section, it is difficult to interpret a result which shows that the children scored negatively on this survey. Clearly, the children may have been saying something about their attitude to speech or they may have been saying something about their speech itself. DeNil and Brutten highlighted this interpretation problem by showing that there was a correlation between stuttering severity scores and survey scores. However, the study definitely suggested that children who have had the disorder for only a short time may feel negative about their speech.

The data which describe children's reactions to stuttering contain some inconsistencies. That is not surprising, considering that they are based on retrospective questionnaire methodology which attempts to record parental impressions of children's feelings. Nonetheless, Johnson et al.'s data consistently indicate that the onset of stuttering has less impact on children than suggested by the Yairi and the Onslow et al. data. But the three studies provide more consistent results about the effect of stuttering on children post onset. Considering this information, along with the fact that early stuttering may appear quite suddenly and be associated with grimacing and body movements (see Part One), it would be difficult to conclude anything but that early stuttering may cause significant distress to young children. It appears, though, that this happens for the minority of children who begin to stutter. Around one fifth of cases of early stuttering may avoid speaking situations, and from around 15 to 30 percent of cases may experience negative feelings—sometimes quite strong—about the problem with their speech.

It is not clear from the research reviewed above whether such negative feelings are chronic, or whether they consist of isolated episodes, as suggested by Bloodstein (1987). And it is not clear whether there is any merit in Van Riper's (1971) suggestion that children with pronounced negative feelings about early stuttering constitute a subgroup of children with the disorder ("Track III"). But it certainly is clear that clinicians need to be aware of the presence of such feelings in this clinical population when making a decision about whether to intervene at the onset of the disorder or at some later time. And of course, for some children, counselling may be necessary about the distress they feel when they begin to stutter.

## Questions about "spontaneous recovery"

Another matter for clinicians to consider in deciding whether to intervene immediately, or to wait for some period of time, is that presently there is much uncertainty about "spontaneous recovery." It is far from clear exactly how many cases will recover by adulthood, with estimates ranging from 30 to 80 percent. And, as mentioned in Part One, it is likely that some—or even all—cases reported recovered actually received intervention from their parents. As Ingham (1983) has noted, it is unreasonable to expect parents to do nothing to assist a child who has begun to stutter. Indeed, careful inspection of the spontaneous recovery literature (Ingham, 1983; Martin & Lindamood, 1986; Wingate, 1976) shows that parents may provide effective operant-like treatments for their children's early stuttering. Recurring reports in this literature are that parents say things such as "stop and start again," "slow down," and "think before you say it" contingent on the stuttering of their children. Onslow, Harrison and Jones (1993) found that 82.8 percent of parents surveyed said that they did such things to help their child stop stuttering. Considering the effectiveness of contingent verbal stimulation in controlling stuttering, and in controlling stuttering in young children in particular (see Part Five), it may be problematic to introduce into clinical practice the notion that there should be no treatment for a period of time. Conceivably, such a practice could remove powerful treatment agents from a stuttering child.

Another query about existing spontaneous recovery estimates is that it is not clear how those estimates relate to a child whom a clinician might encounter in a speech clinic. Much of recovery rate information describes non-clinical populations, which is not necessarily useful in considering whether early stuttering should be treated. The reason for this is that cases of early stuttering who present to a clinic generally may be more severe than nonclinical cases; that might be why they are brought to a clinic. Therefore, those nonclinic cases may be more prone to recovery without formal treatment. It is also the case that there is no agreed way to define, hence diagnose, early stuttering (see Part One). Even in cases where clinicians diagnosed stuttering in this body of literature, it is mostly unclear what procedures they used to do this. But in much of the pertinent literature, diagnoses were not even made by clinicians. For example, Johnson and Associates' (1959) data were based on children who were diagnosed by their parents, and Andrews and Harris (1964) based their data on children diagnosed by "health visitors." These uncertainties and inconsistencies concerning the spontaneous recovery data make it problematic for a clinician to use that data to predict the chance of recovery of any individual, clinically diagnosed case.

### Recovery in the first year after onset:
### The Thousand-Family Study and other data

Another source of help to clinicians about whether to treat immediately or not would be accurate progressive recovery rate data. Such information would inform clinicians of the portion of cases of early stuttering which might recover in a reasonably short period of time. This would enable treatment to be withheld for a certain period after onset with a known chance that a child would recover during that period. Unfortunately, though, it is a lot to ask for such data. A large group of stuttering children would need to be directly observed by clinicians at regular intervals over a long period, and the observations would need to commence at the onset of stuttering. There appears to be only one study which even approximates those methodological qualifications. This is the famous and influential "thousand family study" (Andrews & Harris, 1964, summarized and discussed in Andrews, 1984a).

The study was based on work conducted in 1947 by the University of Durham and the health services of the city of Newcastle-upon-Tyne. The speech development of all children born in the city during May and June that year was studied:

> All of the families were seen regularly by health visitors, who reported on the child's acquisition of speech and her/his progress toward intelligibility, and on the presence of any defects or abnormalities. At regular intervals, speech therapists saw all the children in whom defective speech development or stuttering had been reported, as well as seeing a 1-in-10 sample of the total group. (Andrews, 1984a, pp. 2-3)

At the start of the study there were 1,142 subjects, after 1 year there were 967, and 15 years later at the conclusion of the study there were 763 subjects. Andrews and Harris used the records from this study to identify 43 stuttering subjects; 16 "transient" cases who were affected for less than six months, 18 "remitters" who recovered after being affected for more than six months, and nine "persisting" cases who were still stuttering when the survey concluded. Based on these figures, the reported recovery rate was 79 percent of cases before 16 years of age. But of interest to the present discussion is that 60 percent of the children were reported recovered within the first year after onset, and that Andrews (1984a) cites that figure as a justification for withholding treatment for at least a year.

There is little else in the literature which directly addresses how many recoveries might occur during a 1-year period. Yairi and Ambrose (1992b) reported the first longitudinal study to incorporate direct measures of subjects' stuttering severity. They reported that two of nine clinical cases of early stuttering recovered 12 months after onset without formal treatment.[1] In a report which was survey-based rather than longitudinal, Onslow, Harrison and Jones (1993) presented further data concerning recovery in the first year after onset. They found that 121 children diagnosed as stuttering in a specialist clinic spent an average of 13 months on a waiting list for treatment, during which time parents of 14 children (11.6 percent) reported that their child had recovered and no longer required treatment. An interesting finding in this study was the replication of Johnson and Associates' finding that many parents reported that their children's stuttering was episodic (41.1 percent compared to Johnson et al.'s 34.7 percent). Onslow et al. found that 26 parents reported that their child stopped stuttering while on the waiting list, but a check of clinical records found that 12 of those children had subsequently sought treatment. Again, this substantiates queries about the "thousand family study" finding that many cases recover after a single transient bout of stuttering. It may well be that some cases in that study stuttered episodically for longer periods than reported.

At present, then, there are few reports about how many children will permanently recover from stuttering in the first year after onset, and those reports are conflicting. Andrews and Harris found that a majority will recover, and two other studies found that a minority will recover. One explanation for the discrepancy may be that the Yairi and Ambrose and the Onslow et al. reports underestimated recovery rate in the first year. It is not likely that the former study made errors in assessing individual children, because three

---

[1] Yairi, Ambrose, and Niermann (1993) reported a similar study which followed 16 cases of early stuttering, but only for 6 months. After 6 months, three of these cases met three of the authors' criteria for recovery.

criteria were used for defining recovery, which included a stutter-count measure and a requirement that a parent and clinician agreed that the child was not stuttering. However, Yairi and Ambrose only studied nine children, and such a small sample size may well have underestimated population recovery rate. The Onslow et al. study was based on parents who withdrew their child from a treatment waiting list and did not seek treatment at another clinic. If anything, this study overestimated recovery rate because it was not longitudinal and those recovered children may have begun to stutter again at some later time. Further, both the Yairi and Ambrose and the Onslow et al. studies were likely to have overestimated the number of "clinic-free" recoveries because, at the time of initial assessment, clinicians in both studies gave parents advice about how to handle the stuttering problem. And Onslow et al. reported that 64 percent of the parents who reported intervening with their child's stuttering did so after their initial clinic assessment.

There are good reasons to speculate that Andrews and Harris overestimated with their recovery rate figure of 60 percent in the first year. Those reasons relate to the 16 "transient" cases who stuttered for less than six months. Andrews (1984a) is equivocal about whether those cases should have been diagnosed as stuttering. That reservation is appropriate considering that their presence was detected by nonclinician observers and that the duration of the problem was so short. It certainly seems that such short periods of stuttering do not generally appear in the literature. For example, Ingham (1993) considers that six months of stuttering is a "landmark" for diagnosis of the disorder, and Starkweather, Gottwald, and Halfond (1990) report of their clinic that "a majority of children had been stuttering for 6 to 12 months before our initial contact" (p. 34). Subjects were included in the Onslow, Costa, & Rue's (1990) treatment report only if they had been stuttering for more than 6 months. And the Yale family study (see Part Five) included only cases where stuttering existed for more than 6 months. Additionally, as Ingham (1976) notes, the report on these 16 cases refers to them as "transient nonfluents" rather than "stutterers." If it is accepted that these consider- ations compel that the 16 "transient" cases are removed from Andrews and Harris' data, the recovery rate within one year in that report becomes less than one third.

A recent report by Ramig (1993) is of interest not only because its findings sharply contrast with those mentioned above, but because it fails to support even the notion that many children who begin to stutter will recover without treatment (see Part One). Ramig's report was based on direct speech assessments and long-term follow-up of 21 children who were diagnosed as stuttering but whose parents declined to have their child treated. Five of those children were below 5 years of age at the time of initial assessment. At reassessment, all those five children were found to be stuttering. It is not clear why Ramig's data are so different from other recent data pertaining to recovery from early stuttering. Perhaps the reason relates to the small numbers of subjects who have been studied longitudinally to date. But Ramig's report is a signal that the matter is far from closed.

# The efficiency of treatment services for early stuttering

Andrews (1984a) argues that the substantial recovery rates without formal intervention means that a delay in treatment would improve cost effectiveness. However, withholding treatment for a period of time from young children may not ultimately be more cost efficient, because treatment of advanced stuttering requires much more time than treatment of early stuttering (see Part Three). In particular, if clinicians' reports on the matter are correct, the time consuming problem of posttreatment relapse is much less of a problem with early stuttering than advanced stuttering. At present these impressions are more anecdotal than data based, but if they are confirmed empirically in the future, then it might be a more efficient approach to treat stuttering at its onset rather than to delay treatment for some time. This is particularly so if the delay in treatment were so long that clients reached an age where they could be treated for advanced stuttering in the popular but resource-consuming intensive prolonged-speech formats.

Another consideration is that there are signs that it may be possible to eliminate early stuttering with programs built around verbal RCS. Again, if future research confirms that this is the case, then there will be implications for the cost effectiveness of treatment. As discussed earlier (see Part Three), verbal RCS is a procedure that parents can easily learn to apply in children's everyday speaking environments. In the Onslow, Costa & Rue (1990) study, for instance, the parents of stuttering preschool-age children conducted the treatment under the training and guidance of a clinician. And if the time expenditure in conducting a treatment comes mostly from parents, that treatment becomes appealing in terms of cost efficiency. A preliminary report by Onslow, Andrews, and Lincoln (in press) is pertinent to this matter, because a caseload of early stuttering in that study was treated in a mean of 11.5 clinic sessions. This is far less clinical time than required for instatement of similar treatment effects with adult clients.

Ultimately, the issue of treatment efficiency is linked to the tractability of the disorder. As considered in Part Five, stuttering involves speech motor dysfunction. At some stage in its development stuttering passes out of a stage of being extremely tractable into relative intractability in adulthood. Exactly when stuttering passes across that threshold is far from being known at present, but it is reasonable to speculate that it will be at some time in the life of young speakers when speech motor development is near completion. Therefore, a delay in treatment could cause the disorder to become less tractable (Onslow, 1992; Riley & Riley, 1983; Starkweather, 1990; Starkweather, Gottwald, & Halfond, 1990). It may be the case that a 6-month or 1-year delay in providing treatment is inconsequential. But the imposition of such a delay is a practice that carries an element of doubt.

The issue of the effects of delay on tractability of early stuttering has been addressed in a preliminary empirical report by Starkweather and Gottwald (1993). Fourteen cases of early stuttering were treated with clinical procedures derived from the "demands and capacities model" (see Part Five). Starkweather and Gottwald investigated relations among a number of variables. One variable measured was the amount of time elapsed between stuttering onset and the start of treatment. That variable correlated positively and significantly with the number of treatment sessions required for the children to meet the discharge criteria in the program. In other words, the more time that elapsed after the onset of stuttering, the greater was the number of treatment sessions required.

The authors noted, however, that this and other findings in the study were preliminary and should be qualified. One reason for caution is that there was also a positive, significant correlation between a measure of pretreatment severity and the number of clinic treatment sessions required. This result obscured the meaning of the previous correlation, because it may have been that pretreatment severity was the variable which influenced the duration of treatment. Regression analyses in a large-scale study are required to determine the extent to which a particular variable is able to predict another. Another reservation about Starkweather and Gottwald's results is that early intervention programs typically incorporate a great deal of parental involvement in everyday speaking situations (Starkweather, 1990), and this variable was not accounted for in measures of treatment duration. Finally, correlations in the Starkweather and Gottwald study were small, although significant, and accounted for only a small portion of the variance in the number of treatment sessions required for the children (19 percent). Further research of this kind seems to be potentially profitable. There is little doubt that the period of time from the onset of stuttering to adulthood influences the tractability of the disorder. Research efforts to establish whether that period includes a critical interval shortly after onset may contribute important information about the value of early intervention.

## Conclusions

The withholding of treatment for early stuttering has an underlying assumption that treatment is not required if there is a chance that recovery might eventually occur without it. It is worth noting that such an assumption is uncommon in management practices with other communication disorders. For example, speech pathologists treat children with phonological disorders and specific language impairment, even though eventual recovery from those disorders might occur. There are no grounds to change those practices with the disorder of stuttering.

There is no doubt that a portion of cases of early stuttering recovers without attending a clinic for treatment. Arguably, the data available should be interpreted to mean that the minority of children who begin to stutter will recover within one year after onset. Recovery in many cases is likely to occur because of parental interventions which are initiated either independently or after advice from a speech pathologist. And many children do experience significant distress shortly after stuttering onset.

In light of growing knowledge that early stuttering can be treated effectively in far less than a year—an average of 103 days according to Onslow, Andrews, and Lincoln (1992)—it would be difficult to defend a position that intervention should be withheld for any period of time. Arguably, immediate intervention for a child diagnosed as stuttering is a better strategy than allowing that child to experience a disorder which may be distressing, and which might continue for longer than one year. Immediate intervention is also preferable to assuming that a delay in treatment will not influence the tractability of the disorder. One study has suggested that the period from the onset of stuttering to the start of treatment influences the time taken for treatment (Starkweather & Halfond, 1992). Hence there is an imposing query about a delay in intervention.

In conclusion, the recommendation for treatment not to be withheld from cases of early stuttering could be taken one step further: The notion of an "untreated" case of early stuttering could be abandoned altogether. In reality, such a case may rarely exist. It is certain that parents provide useful assistance to children when they begin to stutter, hence the notion of early stuttering which is "untreated" is misleading. It could be problematic if such misinformation is incorporated within health care services for the disorder, or if it is distributed to parents and health care personnel. Such misinformation has the potential to lead the field back into an era when parents are told to "ignore" early stuttering, as occurred during the apogee of the diagnosogenic theory.

# Part Eight:

# Clinical Issues in Measurement of Stuttering

# Stutter-Count Measures

## Reliability problems

The idea of counting moments of stuttering arose in the 1930s and is generally attributed to Wendell Johnson.[1] That idea opened the disorder to the rigors of scientific enquiry (Bloodstein, 1990), because it became possible to operationalize it. With this tool, an extensive series of investigations began in the University of Iowa during the 1930s.[2] Those investigations foreshadowed much of the measurement techniques used by investigators in subsequent years. Ultimately, measures based on counts of the number of stutters in speech samples assumed a fundamental and accepted place in research and treatment practices for the disorder.

Despite the extensive popularity of stuttering-count measures, it has been well known for a long time that there is something seriously wrong with them! That problem is that independent observers cannot agree very well on the location of stutters. And, as Ingham (in preparation) points out in a summary of the matter, that problem is not resolved when observers are given a definition of stuttering (Curlee, 1981; Martin & Haroldson, 1981; Young, 1975b), or when observers repeat their judgments on a number of occasions (Cordes, Ingham, Frank, & Ingham, 1992; Young, 1975b), or when judges listen to slowed, nondistorted recordings of stuttered speech (Kroll & O'Keefe, 1985; O'Keefe & Kroll, 1980). For some years it was accepted that, despite this problem, observers could generally agree on the total counts of stuttering events in speech samples (Andrews & Ingham 1972; Bloodstein, 1987; Costello & Ingham, 1984a; Ingham, 1984). Ingham (in preparation) has argued that this position arose from reports of satisfactory correlations among judges' total stuttering counts (e.g. Curlee, 1981; Williams, Wark, & Minifie, 1963; Young, 1975b), but those reported correlations often obscured large diferences in judges stuttering counts for individual speech samples.

The problem with reliable counts of stuttering events has been known for half a century. However, it has begun to concern writers recently, with many comments about its serious implications for research and treatment of the disorder (Bloodstein, 1990; Cooper, 1986; Cooper, 1990; Ham, 1989; Hamre, 1992; Ingham, 1990b; Perkins, 1990a; Smith, 1990). It appears that the matter came to a head subsequent to the publication of a study by Kully and Boberg (1988), who collected eight audio tape recordings of stuttered speech and two recordings of nonstuttered speech. These 10 recordings were distributed to 10 clinics throughout the world; Australia, Canada, England and the United States. An experienced clinician from each clinic was instructed to count the number of stuttered syllables on the

---

[1] Van Riper (1992) gives an account of the emergence of this idea, and Johnson (1955) summarizes its development and cites pertinent references.

[2] The appendix to Johnson and Leutenegger (1955) lists all research work, including student theses, completed there until 1954.

tapes.[1] The results were alarming, with substantial differences shown between the clinicians' scores, both in %SS scores and syllables counted. For example, Sample 1 attracted a range of %SS scores from 3.80 to 13.70, and Sample 8 attracted %SS scores ranging from 0 to 4.79. Of particular interest was that the latter sample belonged to a normal speaker! Kully and Boberg pointed out that these interclinic discrepancies are problematic because of what they say about the value of available data that depict outcome evaluation; what should clinicians make of a report that a client's posttreatment stuttering rate is 1 %SS if it is likely another clinic would record a rate of 10 %SS? Even more worrying, what is the clinical significance of any measured posttreatment stuttering rate reduction if a clinician might score normal speech at 4.79 %SS? The Kully and Boberg findings seem not to be spurious, because they were replicated by Ingham and Cordes (1992).

## Conceptual challenges

Bloodstein (1987) has observed that the way something is understood is "intimately bound up with the question of the operations we use to measure it" (p. 2). From that perspective, Johnson's "moment of stuttering" concept can be seen as a way to understand the disorder as episodes of abnormal speech surrounded by normal speech. There have been many challenges to this view of the disorder. One of the first was Williams (1957), who argued that the concept was misguided because, in reality, stuttering was a constant condition rather than a set of discrete speech perturbations. Siegel (1990) suggested that the reliability problems with stuttering indicate that it is time to reconceptualize the disorder; moments of stuttering cannot be counted reliably simply because such moments do not really exist.[2] Stuttering is not a categorical phenomenon that involves discrete moments of speech breakdown, but a continuous phenomenon, where the disorder permeates the person's speech at all times.

If stuttering is a continuous phenomenon, it is easy to understand why moments of stuttering cannot be counted reliably. For the same reason, a group of observers would not be expected to agree about whether a range of temperatures were "hot" or "cold," because the notion of temperature does not contain only those categories, but shows continuous variation. Smith (1990) joins Siegel in arguing that continuous variation is a more justifiable way of viewing stuttering than is categorical partitioning into "stuttered" and "nonstuttered" speech events.

From the perspective of the listener, some writers have suggested that the threshold for perception of a stuttering event depends on several factors. Martin and Haroldson (1981) have suggested that

> a speech perturbation will be identified as a stuttering on the basis of the topography of the speech interruption, the magnitude of the speech interruption, the environment of the speech interruption, and the experiences of the observer. For example, a given observer in a given situation at a given point in time may identify as a stuttering a speech disruption that lasts two seconds, contains a certain amount of force or tension in certain muscle groups, and involves no audible vocalisation. At a different time, or in a different place, or under different

---

[1] Two clinicians counted "syllables disfluent," rather than "syllables stuttered," because that was the usual clinic practice in their clinics.

[2] Although it may be convincing, this is not necessarily the most parsimonious solution to the reliability problem. Hamre (1992) has recently pointed out that it may be difficult for observers to make on-line counts of any events—stuttering or otherwise—that occur during speech. An interesting test of this idea would be for clinicians to determine whether they can agree on the number of times some other event (such as blinking) occurs during speech.

speaking circumstances, or when listening to a different speaker, the observer's threshold for identifying stuttering may be different and that same observer would not identify the same behaviors as stuttering. (p. 62)

Smith (1990) shares this view by stating that stuttering is perceived "when processes underlying speech breakdown converge to disrupt speech production in a manner that the individual and his culture regard as abnormal"(p. 399). Adams and Runyan (1981) have considered the matter from the perspective of the speaker, by speculating that "all the composite physiologic, aerodynamic, and temporal values generated by the respiratory, phonatory, and articulatory systems" (p. 205) can be considered together as responsible for stuttering, where

> stuttering and fluency are viewed as events along a continuum, so that as speech flows forward there is a drift, sometimes gradual, sometimes rapid, toward stuttering. The closer a speaker comes to that overt stutttering event, the more abnormal the speech produced, and the more perceptibly different the speech fluency. Similarly, after stuttering has occurred, there is a relatively gradual return toward normal fluency. During this post-stuttering transition, subtle anomalies are still present in the speech signal . (Adams & Runyan, 1981, p. 205)

One development from these ideas is that stuttering and normal disfluency lie on opposite ends of a continuum. Siegel (personal communication, 1993) has gone as far as suggesting that the restructuring of concepts of the disorder should include abandoning the distinction between stuttering and normal disfluency, and accepting that stuttering can occur in any speaker, just as normal disfluencies can. In support of this argument, Siegel notes that it is common in health care to conceptualise pathological conditions as laying along a continuum. For example, anxiety is a common experience of everyday life, but it also can amount to a pathological condition. Smith (1990) seems to concur, stating that the notion of stuttering as a continuous phenomenon implies that factors which increase the "probability of speech breakdown in stuttering...also would increase the likelihood of disfluent speech in nonstutterers" (p. 399). Borden (1990) has pointed out that stuttering and normal disfluency may be perceived as laying on a continuum even though, in reality, they may be two distinct physiological states. In other words, stuttering and normal disfluency may to some extent look similar even though they have different causes.

There has been some research directed at the issue of whether or not stuttering is a continuous problem for a speaker. Wendahl and Cole (1961) tested the matter in a study where they assembled a stimulus tape containing 64 sentences which were read by eight stuttering subjects and eight nonstuttering subjects. Stutters were deleted from the recordings of the stuttering subjects, and matching deleted segments were edited from the recordings of the control subjects. When this stimulus tape was presented to a group of listeners, Wendahl and Cole reported that the listeners were able to determine which samples were from the stuttering subjects and which samples were from the nonstuttering subjects. This result proved to be quite controversial when Young (1964) replicated the experiment, using Wendahl and Cole's stimulus tape, but with what were claimed to be some methodological improvements in obtaining listeners' responses. Further, Young utilized a statistical analysis procedure that was claimed to be more appropriate to the experiment. Young's results were the opposite to those of Wendahl and Cole. Listeners were unable to distinguish, beyond levels expected by chance, between the stutter-free speech of experimental subjects and the speech of control subjects.

Subsequently, Few and Lingwall (1977) showed that 10-second stutter-free speech samples from 14 stuttering subjects could not be distinguished by listeners from the speech of nonstuttering controls. A study by Brown and Colcord (1987) produced a different result. Brown and Colcord used stutter-free speech segments from seven stuttering subjects with a mean age of 14 years 8 months, and the speech of matched controls. Using a stimulus-pair judgement procedure, it was determined that only two of the stuttering subjects could not be identified by listeners.[1] Krikorian and Runyan (1983) reported a study with similar methodology to Wendahl and Cole, but with 15 stuttering subjects with a mean age of 5 years 3 months. It was reported that listeners were unable to separate the stuttering children from controls at a level that exceeded chance expectation. That result was repeated by Colcord and Gregory (1987) with nine stuttering children, of mean age 6 years 8 months, and their matched controls. The children's speech samples consisted of stutter-free sentences, and listeners were asked to respond both with a forced-choice and stimulus-pair judgement paradigm. Overall, results indicated that listeners were unable to determine which were the stuttering children and which were the controls.

On balance, these perceptual studies generally seem to support Johnson's "moment of stuttering" by showing that the stutter-free speech of those who stutter is perceptually normal. However, these results are contradicted by a body of findings showing that the stutter-free speech of people who stutter differs from normal speakers (see page 182). How, then, should these contradictory findings be reconciled? One tempting conclusion is that the stutter-free speech of people who stutter indeed does contain unusual features, but those unusual features cannot be perceived by listeners. This conclusion might be thought reasonable because it is quite conceivable that some acoustic differences are not apparent perceptually. In the body of research concerned, the differences that have been detected are small and unlikely to be detected by listeners. Further, the differences mostly relate to durations of speech events such as vowel duration and voice onset time. However, the durations of such events vary dramatically within a subject according to numerous parameters, including articulatory context and position within an utterance. So it is quite likely that differences in mean acoustic measures in stuttered speech would not be detectable when listening to the speaker.

## Clinical implications

In summary, then, there have been serious conceptual challenges to the notion of stuttering as a series of categorical events. Those challenges are substantiated by research findings that stutter-free speech contains unusual features, and by findings that stutters cannot be counted reliably. It would be difficult to validly conceptualize the disorder as a set of categorical speech perturbations. On first consideration, this might seem to be a situation with fearsome implications for clinical management. Should clinicians abandon the concept of a moment of stuttering and cease to use stutter-count measures in clinical practice? Certainly not, because the concept of a moment of stuttering is enormously useful to clinicians and it can continue to be so, providing the convenience does not lead to a belief that stuttering really does consist of discrete events (G.M. Siegel, personal communication, 1992).

The matter of reliability of stuttering counts carries the most serious clinical implications, because they suggest that the foundation of clinical practice might be shaky (Ingham, 1990b). The seriousness of such a prospect compels that it is carefully considered. Before considering the issue of reliability, though, it is important to consider the notion of

---

[1] These studies do not specify the treatment histories of their subjects. Several do not mention the treatment history of their subjects (Brown and Colcord, 1987; Krikorian and Runyan, 1983; Wendahl & Cole, 1961), and two indicate only that their subjects were receiving treatment when the study was conducted (Colcord & Gregory, 1987; Few & Lingwall, 1972). This is a problem because any subjects in those studies who were using a speech-pattern could have been identified because of that speech pattern.

reliability itself. If systematic behavioral data trends are detected by an observer, there are two possible explanations. The first is that the variation is due to change in the behavior in question. But the second explanation is that the variation is due to the observer. The point of reliability assessment is to demonstrate that the effects reported are due to change in the variable being measured, not to variation arising from the observer. This view suggests that it is meaningless to think about reliability of data measures independently of the size of the effect that those measures purport to detect.

In the field of stuttering treatment, most effect sizes are large because sizeable reductions in stuttering severity are needed for clinical significance. Now, consider data that are reliable to the extent that observers might have made observational errors causing variation across 30 percent of the measurement scale. Imagine a result where Condition A has a mean score of 80 %SS and Condition B has a mean score of 20 %SS. The extent of reliability of the data means that we can be confident that actual scores in Condition A are somewhere in the range 95-65 %SS and the actual scores in Condition B are somewhere in the range 35-5 %SS. The ranges do not overlap, so we still can be sure that an effect is present.[1] Consider the Howie, Tanner, and Andrews (1981) report of treatment effects for 79 subjects (see Part Four), where means of 13.8 %SS pretreatment and 3.1 %SS posttreatment were reported. Applying the above reasoning, the data in such a study could vary capriciously across 10 percent of the %SS scale without impairing the capacity of the study to detect the effect size.[2]

Another perspective on the reliability of speech measures is that it cannot be evaluated without reference to the purpose of those measures. There is no doubt that observers cannot agree on the total number of stutters in speech samples, and that they cannot reliably determine where stutters are located in speech samples. But that is not the major issue in clinical practice. In clinical practice, the purpose of collecting speech measures is to document trends in speech performance from before to after treatment, or during treatment. This point is illustrated in Figure 10, which is a re-arrangement of the Kully and Boberg (1988) data collected by the eight clinicians who counted stutters. Figure 10 shows clearly that these clinicians, although showing disparate %SS scores, generally identified the same data trends nonetheless. For example, all clinicians recorded a substantial difference between Sample 3 and Sample 5. So, the Kully and Boberg data actually might be interpreted as support for the capacity of different clinicians to reliably use a stutter-count measure to document trends in speech performance.

Even so, this does not negate the problem that observers may not be able to reliably count the number of stutters present in speech samples. If research is concerned with the number of stutters in speech samples, then reliability problems with that measure are a serious threat to the value of that research. Further, a great deal of stuttering research depends on isolating speech samples which are free of stuttering. An example of this is research into the perceptual and acoustic features of stutter-free speech mentioned above. If stuttering events cannot be identified reliably, then the confidence in such research findings is reduced. However, these matters do not pose such a problem for clinicians, because stuttering counts are only a part of the information that allows them to evaluate and document the progress of their treatments. Expert clinicians base their treatment decisions

---

[1] In contrast, speech training for prelinguistically profoundly hearing impaired children is a different matter altogether. There, a 5 percent improvement in intelligibility is clinically significant, and therefore reliability requirements would be more stringent.

[2] This argument assumes that the study was sufficiently well controlled to prevent the occurence of any systematic observer bias. For example, it is assumed that observers who generated the %SS scores were unaware of whether each sample was pretreatment or posttreatment.

on various kinds of information; client reports of speech performance and satisfaction, other kinds of speech measures such as severity and naturalness ratings, their own judgement about whether the client's speech resembles normal speech, reports of significant others in the client's environment, and so on. No clinician would depend solely on stutter-count measures for information about clients' speech performance.

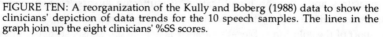

FIGURE TEN: A reorganization of the Kully and Boberg (1988) data to show the clinicians' depiction of data trends for the 10 speech samples. The lines in the graph join up the eight clinicians' %SS scores.

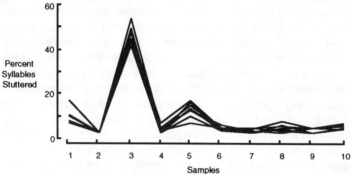

It is also worth noting that most of the research into reliability of stuttering counts does not bear directly on the value of stuttering counts made by clinicians in day-to-day clinical practice. It may be the case that a group of clinicians shows poor agreement on how many stutters are in speech samples, such as in studies by Kully and Boberg (1988) and Ingham and Cordes (1992). But clinicians in those studies listened only to short speech samples from clients, whereas clinicians have many hours of extended personal contact with clients. It is possible that clinicians, under those circumstances, would agree on the number of stutters in clients' speech. In other words, if an experiment was conducted where a group of clinicians each established a clinical relationship with clients, it is conceivable that they might agree on the number of stutters contained in that person's speech samples.

Although interjudge reliability is an important issue, another issue in the value of clinicians' stuttering counts is intrajudge reliability. Arguably, the most critical reliability concern for clinicians is to be internally consistent from session to session in how many stutters they count in the speech of clients, and to be internally consistent in what they judge is a stutter in a client's speech. This is especially the case during clinical trials when a client speaks and the clinician provides feedback when stuttering occurs. In an established clinical relationship with a client, clinicians may have no problems with intrajudge reliability. Packman, Ingham and Onslow (1993) recently confirmed that this may be the case. A group of seven clinicians who worked in one clinic counted stutters in speech samples. As expected, the clinicians showed considerable discrepancies in the number of stutters counted in the speech samples. But when they were asked to repeat the experimental task some time later, the clinicians showed impressive levels of intrajudge agreement. So those clinicians, although not agreeing about the number of stutters in clients' samples, were clearly capable of making consistent clinical measures and providing feedback about stuttering events to their clients.

Siegel (1990) has made an interesting observation about the research which has consistently found poor reliability for stuttering counts. He points out that such measures have been used as a basis for the consistent reporting of so many effects associated with the disorder. For example, hundreds of reports have documented the adaptation effect, the responsiveness of stuttering to operant methodology, and reduced stuttering in posttreatment speech samples. How could those results have been obtained if the measures in those reports were intrinsically unreliable? In fact, Siegel argues, such replication is arguably the strongest test of reliability (Sidman, 1960). Siegel's paradox might also be applied to stuttering treatment: Most behaviorally-based treatments depend on stuttering-count measures and clinician identification of stuttering events, so how can clinicians conduct those treatments if stutters cannot be counted or identified reliably?

One part of the solution to Siegel's paradox is that, in one sense, stutter-count measures are not unreliable at all. The literature concerning conditions and treatments which control stuttering depends on the use of stuttering counts to detect data trends. And, as argued above, there is every reason to believe that clinicians can use such measures to perform that function reliably. Siegel (1990) has offered another potential solution to his paradox. One of these concerns the notion of "kernel" and "accessory" stuttering behaviors (Wingate, 1964). This idea has been reiterated several times (for example, Brutten & Shoemaker, 1967; Van Riper, 1971). It amounts to a position that stuttering fundamentally consists of repetitions, blocks, and prolongations, and all the other countless behaviors of stuttering are the speaker's struggle with the condition, or attempts to control or conceal it. Siegel suggests that it may be the "accessory" behaviors of stuttering which cause all the trouble with reliabilty. Perhaps the "kernel" stutters are easy to identify, and are generally identified and counted reliably, but attempts to count the "accessory" behaviors spoil reliability. This would explain why research has shown that RCS can control stuttering and also that stuttering events cannot be counted reliably; perhaps it is only the "core" behaviors which need to receive the contingent stimulation for the control of stuttering.

In summary, Johnson's "moment of stuttering" has been one of the most productive ideas in the history of this field. It is difficult to imagine that its controversial nature will ever outweigh its convenience and usefulness for clinicians. That convenience, though, is obtained at the cost of nagging problems with reliability. Those problems are not as directly damaging to clinical practice as they are to research into the disorder. But ultimately those problems may affect clinical practice if they impede clinical research. In attempting to resolve the reliability problems in the field, Ingham and colleages (Cordes, Ingham, Frank, & Ingham, 1992; Ingham, Cordes, & Gow, 1993; ) are investigating the possibility that stutter-count measures based on intervals might be a way to resolve this crisis. It may prove to be the case that observers can be trained to reliably count the number of short intervals that do and do not contain stuttering.

# Measures of Attitude and Control

## Attitude to communication

Erickson (1969) developed a 39-item questionnaire which was designed to measure the attitudes about communication held by people who stutter. Erickson presented a list of questionnaire responses which were typical of people who stutter, and responses typical of nonstuttering speakers. Respondents are required to respond "true" or "false" to each item, and a point is scored for a response typical of someone who stutters, and the total score is taken as an indication of the extent to which the respondent has attitudes about communication which are typical of someone who stutters. Andrews and Cutler (1974) had a group of stuttering subjects, and also a group of normal speakers, complete Erickson's scale during the course of treatment. Questionnaire items that were shown to be unreliable or invalid were deleted, reducing the original to a 24-item scale. This scale developed by Andrews and Cutler has become known as the S24 scale. Examples of items to which responses of "true" or "false" are elicited are as follows: "I often ask questions at group discussions," "I talk better than I write," and "I often feel nervous when talking."

In a second part of their study, Andrews and Cutler measured the speech performance of another group of stuttering subjects before, during and after a prolonged-speech treatment program. Responses on the S24 scale closely reflected speech performance. Attitude to communication scores improved following the instatement part of the program, but reached scores equivalent to normal speakers only after the completion of the transfer part of the program. These results introduced the idea that normalization of communication attitudes is an important component of stuttering treatment.

Guitar (1976) investigated whether any pretreatment measures could predict treatment outcome. In an initial study, a variety of stuttering-count and non-behavioral measures were obtained for a group of clients pretreatment and one year following treatment. These measures included the S24 scale, along with measures of neuroticism and extroversion. Many significant correlations were found between pretreatment and posttreatment measures. A regression analysis was conducted to predict posttreatment outcome from pretreatment measures. The S24 scale was identified as the best single predictor of treatment outcome, which added to the considerable importance of the findings of Andrews and Cutler. In a second group of treatment clients, Guitar used multiple regression analysis to predict treatment outcome. It was reported that pretreatment measures on the S24 scale were a useful predictor of treatment outcome.

The findings outlined above were added to by an influential study by Guitar and Bass (1978). Twenty clients completed the S24 scale before, immediately after, and one year after an intensive treatment program. Measures of %SS were obtained pretreatment and at one year posttreatment. On the basis of immediate posttreatment S24 scores, subjects were partitioned into two groups with different communication attitudes. These two groups were a "normalized" and "nonnormalized group." The former group showed S24 scores similar to those achieved by normal speakers, and the latter group did not. Results showed that the normalized group of clients had significantly better %SS scores at one year posttreatment.

Guitar and Bass concluded that normalization of communication attitude during the treatment process increased the chance of long-term success in treatment.

## Locus of control

The concept of locus of control concerns the extent to which people feel that they can influence what happens to them. An "external" locus of control is where a person feels helpless in controlling life, and an "internal" locus of control indicates that someone feels empowered to influence the course of life events. Craig and Howie (1982) speculated that these ideas might be pertinent to stuttering treatment, because clients who have an internal locus of control might take responsibility to do the things their treatment program taught them to do in order not to stutter. Craig and Howie used a scale developed by Rotter (1966) to measure the pretreatment locus of control of 30 clients in a prolonged-speech treatment program, and again at 18 months posttreatment. They reported a moderate correlation between the change in locus of control scores over the pretreatment-posttreatment period and the change in %SS scores over the same period.

Subsequently, Craig, Franklin, & Andrews (1984) developed a scale designed specifically "to measure the extent to which subjects perceive responsibility for their personal problem behavior" (p. 174). The scale consisted of 17 statements, such as "a great deal of what happens to me is just a matter of chance," "I believe a person can really be the master of his fate," and "I am confident of being able to deal successfully with future problems." This scale allowed respondents a choice of six responses to each item, ranging from "strongly disagree" to "strongly agree." In order to assess the validity of this scale, Craig et al. assessed whether it could distinguish between people with chronic conditions and control subjects. They administered their scale to a group of stuttering subjects and a group of agrophobic subjects, and also to two control groups. Results showed that the experimental subjects scored higher (more "external" locus of control) than the controls. Craig et al. then conducted a further study of 45 clients in a prolonged speech treatment program. They divided those clients into a group of 32 who relapsed (more than 2 %SS during an 10-months posttreatment assessment) and a group of 13 who did not relapse (less than 2 %SS on the same measure). Results showed that a reduced (internalized) locus of control score was associated with less chance of relapse, and that an unchanged or increased (externalized) score was associated with more chance of relapse. Craig and Andrews (1985) replicated the Craig, Franklin, and Andrews (1984) finding that long-term outcome relates to changes in locus of control scores. They conducted measures on 17 subjects pretreatment, posttreatment and 10 months posttreatment. Fourteen subjects "internalized" their locus of control, and only two of those relapsed (greater than 2 %SS 10 months posttreatment). Three subjects did not "internalize" locus of control, and each of those subjects relapsed.

## Clinical implications and issues

The notion of locus of control and, especially, attitude to communication seem to be popular ones. Several scales exist which pertain to attitude to communication, such as the "Perceptions of Stuttering Inventory" (Woolf, 1967), the "Stutterer's Self Ratings of Reactions to Speech Situations" the "Iowa Scale of Attitude Toward Stuttering" (Johnson, Darley, & Spriestersbach, 1953), and the "Reaction to Self-Descriptive Statments" (Prins, 1993). The report by DeNil and Brutten (1991) mentioned on page 192 incorporated a "Children's Attitude Test," and Peters and Guitar (1991) describe an "A-19" scale for assessing children's communication attitudes. One likely reason for the popularity of these scales is a perception of the importance of communication attitude in stuttering treatment. It is obvious that clients need to be positive about their capacity to communicate effectively, and that they need to take responsibility for their treatment in order to succeed. No clinician would fail to address problems in either of these areas with clients. Nor would a clinician be likely to overlook the possibility that people who stutter may have poor attitudes to communication and may feel that they are helpless to control their speech, as the studies mentioned above and others (DeNil & Brutten, 1991; Miller & Watson, 1992; Watson, 1988) have verified.

Attitude and locus of control have raised some controversy in the literature (Finn & Gow, 1989; Ingham, 1979; Guitar, 1979; Ulliana & Ingham; 1984; Young, 1981). That controversy does not relate the clinical importance of those constructs; it relates to the conclusions from studies which deal with them. One issue arises from the fact that claims about the attitude and locus of control measures are based on correlations between those measures and posttreatment measures of speech performance. One interpretation of correlation is that the two variables are discrete and that they covary, but another interpretation is that the two variables are in reality the same thing.

Ulliana and Ingham (1984) presented a conceptual and experimental challenge to the S24 scale along these lines. Items on the S24 scale refer to speaking situations, and they raised the possibility that responses to those items might reflect speech behavior rather than attitude to speech. For example, people who respond "no" to the question "I face most speaking situations with complete confidence" could simply be saying that their speech is poor in most situations. Another way of saying this is that there may be some question about the relative contribution of behavioral (stuttering) and nonbehavioral (attitude) factors in S24 responses. The first part of the Ulliana and Ingham study addressed whether the S24 scale measures attitudes to speech rather than speech behavior. The scale was administered to 19 stuttering subjects weekly for 3 weeks. Along with each S24 response, subjects indicated whether their response was governed by speech behavior or attitudes and feelings, or neither. Results showed that attitudes and feelings influenced responses, but mostly responses were influenced by behavioral considerations.

Responses on the S24 scale typical of stuttering speakers are referred to as scored responses, and responses typical of nonstuttering speakers are referred to as nonscored responses. The second part of the Ulliana and Ingam study involved three subjects from the first part of the study who consistently nominated a certain situation as the basis of a scored and an unscored response to an S24 item. Each of these three subjects then tape recorded their speech in the nominated situations weekly for 6 weeks. Results showed that each of the subjects had a lower stuttering severity in the nonscored situation than in the scored situation. In other words, they stuttered less in situations in which the S24 scale suggested that their attitude to communication was good, and they stuttered more in situations where the S24 scale suggested that attitude to communication was poor. Ulliana and Ingham argued that these data queried whether the S24 scale measures something independent of speech behavior.

The problematic nature of research into the role of attitude and control in posttreatment relapse is exemplified in a report by Andrews and Craig (1988). They studied relapse in 84 clients and whether or not those clients had achieved three treatment goals at the end of their prolonged-speech program. The treatment goals were (1) being able to speak with zero stuttering, (2) an internalized locus of control, and (3) normalized attitude to communication. Relapse was defined as more than 2 %SS during a 600-syllable telephone call to a stranger 10-18 months after the conclusion of the program. Craig and Andrews reported that the success rate of the clients related systematically to how many of the treatment goals were achieved, and that 97 percent of the clients who had achieved all three of the treatment goals did not relapse.

This report implies that, in order to solve the problem of posttreatment relapse, all clinicians need do is to have clients achieve stutter-free speech, an internalized locus of control, and normalized atttitude to communication. This seems to be a simplification of a complex matter. Some idea of its complexity can be obtained by contemplating a few variables pertaining to clients, apart from control and attitude, which might contribute to posttreatment relapes. These variables have been mentioned in Parts Two and Four. For example, a client may relapse because of insufficient time or motivation to complete the regular practice required to maintain stutter free speech. Alternatively, the client may be practicing prolonged speech regularly, but inadvertently practicing errors in speech skills such as "soft contacts" or "gentle onsets." Or perhaps the client never learned those speech skills well enough in the first place to control stuttering for a long period of time. Or a client may relapse simply because the benefits achieved from stutter-free speech do not seem to be worth the effort of continual attention to speech. It is even possible that clients will relapse because stuttered speech was never really part of their presenting complaint in the first place. Alternatively, the client's speech may feel or sound unnatural, or debilitating anxiety in speaking situations may disrupt the use of the new speech pattern.

The above list could continue, but that is not the point here. The point is that part of being a successful clinician is being able to prevent relapse by foreseeing factors which might cause it and by planning treatments accordingly. Another part of being a clinician is accepting the limitations of that role. One such limitation is that there is much yet to know about posttreatment relapse, and much work yet to be done to resolve the problem. It is a problematic belief that internalized locus of control and attitude change are an adequate insight into the problem and a complete clinical defence against it. That belief could have the effect of diverting clinicians' attention from other obvious contributions to the problem. Even worse, it might have the effect that the victims of stuttering will be blamed for failed treatments (A. Packman, personal communication, 1993). It would not be productive for clinicians to believe that they have perfect treatments and that if those treatments fail, then the client is at fault and needs to improve in attitude to communication and sense of control over the problem of stuttering.

# References

Adams, M.R. (1977). A clinical strategy for differentiating the normally nonfluent child and the incipient stutterer. *Journal of Fluency Disorders, 2,* 141-148.

Adams, M.R. (1984). The differential assessment and direct treatment of stuttering. In J. Costello (Ed.), *Speech disorders in children.* San Diego: College-Hill Press.

Adams, M.R. (1985). The speech physiology of stutterers: Present status. *Seminars in Speech and Language, 6,* 177-196.

Adams, M.R. (1987). Voiced onsets and segment durations of normal speakers and beginning stutterers. *Journal of Fluency Disorders, 12,* 133-139.

Adams, M.R. (1990). The demands and capacities model I: Theoretical elaborations. *Journal of Fluency Disorders, 15,* 135-141.

Adams, M.R., Freeman, F.J., & Conture, E.G. (1984) Laryngeal dynamics of stutterers. In R.F. Curlee & W.H. Perkins (Eds.), *Nature and treatment of stuttering: New directions.* San Diego: College-Hill Press.

Adams, M.R., & Runyan, C.M. (1981). Stuttering and fluency: Exclusive events or points on a continuum? *Journal of Fluency Disorders, 6,* 197-218.

Ainsworth, S., & Fraser, J. (1987). *If your child stutters: A guide for parents* (2nd. Ed.). Memphis: Speech Foundation of America.

Andrews, C., Webber, M., Costa, L., Harrison, E., Onslow, M., & Packman , A. (1992). Less pain, how much gain? Generalization and maintenance from a one-day prolonged-speech instatement procedure for stuttering. Paper presented at the *Annual Conference of the Australian Association of Speech and Hearing,* Melbourne, February.

Andrews, G. & Craig, A. (1988). Prediction of outcome after treatment for stuttering. *British Journal of Psychiatry, 153,* 236-240.

Andrews, G. (1984a). Epidemiology of stuttering. In R.F. Curlee and W.H. Perkins (Eds.), *Nature and treatment of stuttering: New directions .* San Diego: College-Hill Press.

Andrews, G. (1984b). Evaluation of the benefits of treatment. In W. H. Perkins (Ed.), *Stuttering disorders .* New York: Thieme-Stratton.

Andrews, G., & Craig, A. (1988). Prediction of outcome after treatment for stuttering. *British Journal of Psychiatry, 153,* 236-240.

Andrews, G., Craig, A., Feyer, A.M., Hoddinott, S., Howie, P., & Neilson, M. (1983). Stuttering: A review of research findings and theories circa 1982. *Journal of Speech and Hearing Disorders, 48,* 226-246.

Andrews, G., & Cutler, J. (1974). Stuttering therapy: The relation between changes in symptom level and attitudes. *Journal of Speech and Hearing Disorders, 39,* 312-319.

Andrews, G., & Feyer, A. M. (1985). Does behaviour therapy still work when the experimenters have departed? *Behavior Modification, 9,* 443-456.

Andrews, G., Guitar, B., & Howie, P. (1980). Meta-analysis of the effects of stuttering treatment. *Journal of Speech and Hearing Disorders, 45,* 287-307.

Andrews, G., & Harris, M. (1964). *The syndrome of stuttering.* Clinics in Developmental Medicine, No. 17. London: Heinemann.

Andrews, G., & Ingham, R.J. (1972). An approach to the evaluation of stuttering therapy. *Journal of Speech and Hearing Research, 15,* 296-302.

Andrews, G., Morris-Yates, A, Howie, P., Martin, N. (1991). Genetic factors in stuttering confirmed. *Archives of General Psychiatry, 48,* 1034-1035.

Andrews, G., Neilson, M., & Cassar, M. (1987). Informing stutterers about treatment. In L. Rustin, H. Purser, & D. Rowley (Eds.), *Progress in the treatment of fluency disorders.* London: Taylor & Francis.

ASHA (1990). Let's talk. *ASHA, June/July, 63.*

Attanasio, J. (1991). Research design issues in relationships between anxiety and stuttering: Comments on Craig (1990). *Journal of Speech and Hearing Research, 34,* 1079-1080.

Australian Speak Easy Association (1986). *The young stutterer* (Film). Lismore, Australia: Image North Television Productions.

Baer, D. (1988). If you know why you're changing a behavior, you'll know when you've changed it enough. *Behavioral Assessment, 10,* 219-223.

Baer, D. (1990). The critical issue in treatment efficacy is knowing why treatment was applied: A student's response to Roger Ingham. In L.B. Olswang, C.K. Thompson, S. Warren, & N.J. Minghetti, (Eds.), *Treatment efficacy research in communication disorders*. Rockville, MD: American Speech-Language-Hearing Foundation .

Barlow, D.H., & Hersen, M. (1984). *Single case experimental designs: Strategies for studying behavior change* (2nd Ed.). New York: Pergamon Press.

Bellack, A.S., & Hersen, M. (1977) *Behavior modification: An introductory textbook*. New York: Oxford University Press.

Bjerkan, B. (1980). Word fragmentations and repetitions in the spontaneous speech of 2-6-year-old children. *Journal of Fluency Disorders, 5,* 137-148.

Block, S.L., & Ingham, R.J. (1983). A quantitative analysis of the effects of the Edinburgh Masker on stuttering: Some preliminary findings. *Proceedings of the XIXth congress of the International Association of Logopaedics and Phoniatrics.*

Bloodstein, O. (1961). The development of stuttering: III. Theoretical and clinical implications. *Journal of Speech and Hearing Disorders, 26,* 67-82.

Bloodstein, O. (1975). Stuttering as tension and fragmentation. In J. Eisenson (Ed.), *Stuttering: A second symposium* . New York: Harper and Row.

Bloodstein, O. (1984). Stuttering as an anticipatory struggle disorder. In R.F. Curlee and W.H. Perkins (Eds.), *Nature and treatment of stuttering: New directions* . San Diego: College-Hill Press.

Bloodstein, O. (1986). Semantics and beliefs. In G.H. Shames and H. Rubin (Eds.), *Stuttering then and now* . Columbus: Charles E. Merrill.

Bloodstein, O. (1987) *A handbook on stuttering* (4th Ed.). Chicago: National Easter Seal Society.

Bloodstein, O. (1990). On pluttering, skivvering, and floggering: A commentary. *Journal of Speech and Hearing Disorders, 55,* 392-393.

Bloodstein, O., & Grossman, M. (1981). Early stutterings: Some aspects of their form and distribution. *Journal of Speech and Hearing Research, 24,* 298-302.

Bluemel, C.S. (1932). Primary and secondary stammering. *Quarterly Journal of Speech, 18,* 187-200.

Boberg, E. (1980). Intensive adult therapy program. *Seminars in Speech, Language, and Hearing, 1,* 365-373.

Boberg, E. (1981). Maintenance of fluency: An experimental program. In E. Boberg (Ed.), *Maintenance of fluency*. New York: Elsevier.

Boberg, E. (1986). Relapse and outcome. In G. H. Shames & H. Rubin (Eds.), *Stuttering then and now* . Columbus: Charles E. Merrill.

Boberg, E., Howie, P., & Woods, L. (1979). Maintenance of fluency: A review. *Journal of Fluency Disorders, 4,* 93-116.

Boberg, E., & Kully, D. (1985). *Comprehensive stuttering treatment program* . San Diego: College-Hill Press.

Boberg, E., & Sawyer, L. (1977). The maintenance of fluency following intensive therapy. *Human Communication, 2,* 21-28.

Boberg, E., Yeudall, L. T., Schopflocher, D., & Bo-Lassen, P. (1983). The effect of an intensive behavioral program on the distribution of EEG alpha power in stutterers during the processing of verbal and visuospatial information. *Journal of Fluency Disorders, 8,* 245-263.

Borden, G.J. (1990). Subtyping adult stutterers for research purposes. *ASHA Reports, 18,* 58-62.

Borden, G.J., Baer, T., & Kenney, M.K. (1985). Onset of voicing in stuttered and fluent utterances. *Journal of Speech and Hearing Research, 28,* 363-372.

Borden, G.J., Kim, D.H., & Spiegler, K. (1987). Acoustics of stop consonant-vowel relationships during fluent and stuttered utterances. *Journal of Fluency Disorders, 12,* 175-184.

Borman, E.G. (1969). "Ephphatha, or, some advice to stammerers." Journal of Speech and Hearing Research, 12, 453-461.

Brown, S.I., & Colcord, R.D. (1987). Perceptual comparisons of adolescent stutterers' and nonstutterers' fluent speech. *Journal of Fluency Disorders, 12,* 419-427.

Browning, R. (1967). Behavior therapy for stuttering in a schizophrenic child. *Behaviour Research and Therapy, 5,* 27-35.

Brutten, G.J. (1983). A reply to Costello and (Roemer) Hurst. *Journal of Speech and Hearing Research, 26,* 155-156.

Brutten, G.J., & Shoemaker, D.J. (1971) A two-factor learning theory of stuttering. In L.E. Travis (Ed.), *Handbook of speech pathology and audiology*. New York: Appleton-Century-Crofts.

Burke, B. (1973). The identification and measurement of stuttering in real time: The Prince Henry Yardstick. *Australian Journal of Human Communication Disorders, 1,* 42-43.

Camarata, S.M., (1989). Final consonant repetition: A linguistic perspective. *Journal of Speech and Hearing Disorders, 54,* 159-162.

Clark, R.M. (1964). Our enterprising predecessors and Charles Sydney Bluemel. *Asha, 6,* 107-114.

Colburn, N. (1985). Clustering of disfluency in nonstuttering childrens' early utterances. *Journal of Fluency Disorders, 10,* 51-58.

Colcord, R.D., & Gregory, H.H. (1987). Perceptual analyses of stuttering and nonstuttering children's fluent speech. *Journal of Fluency Disorders, 12,* 185-195.

Conture, E. (1982). *Stuttering.* Englewood Cliffs, N.J.: Prentice Hall.

Conture, E. (1990). *Stuttering* (2nd. Ed.). Englewood Cliffs, N.J.: Prentice Hall.

Conture, E.G., & Caruso, A.J. (1987). Assessment and diagnosis of childhood dysfluency. In L. Rustin, H. Purser, & D. Rowley (Eds.), *Progress in the treatment of fluency disorders.* London: Taylor and Francis.

Conture, E., & Kelly, E. (1991). Young stutterers' nonspeech behaviors during stuttering. *Journal of Speech and Hearing Research, 34,* 1041-1056.

Conture, E.G., Rothenberg, M., & Molitor, R.D. (1986). Electroglottographic observations of young stutterers' fluency. *Journal of Speech and Hearing Research, 29,* 384-393.

Cooper, E.B. (1986). Treatment of disfluency: Future trends. *Journal of Fluency Disorders, 11,* 317-327.

Cooper, E.B. (1987). The Chronic Perseverative Stuttering Syndrome; incurable stuttering. *Journal of Fluency Disorders, 12,* 381-388.

Cooper, E.B., & Cooper, C S. (1985). Clinician attitudes toward stuttering: A decade of change (1973-1983). *Journal of Fluency Disorders, 10,* 19-33.

Cooper, E.B., & Rustin, L. (1985). Clinician attitudes towards stuttering in the United States and Great Britain: A cross-cultural study. *Journal of Fluency Disorders, 10,* 1-17.

Cooper, E.G. (1987). The Cooper personalized fluency control therapy. In L. Rustin, H. Purser, and D. Rowley (Eds.), *Progress in the treatment of fluency disorders .* London: Taylor and Francis.

Cooper, J.A. (1990). Research directions in stuttering: Consensus and conflict. *ASHA Reports, 18,* 98-100.

Coppola, V.A., & Yairi, E. (1982). Rhythmic speech training with preschool stuttering children: An experimental study. *Journal of Fluency Disorders, 7,* 447-457.

Cordes, A.K., Ingham, R.J, Frank, P., & Ingham, J.C. (1992). Time interval analysis of interjudge and intrajudge agreement for stuttering event judgements. *Journal of Speech and Hearing Research, 35,* 483-494.

Costello, J. (1975). The establishment of fluency with time-out procedures: Three case studies. *Journal of Speech and Hearing Disorders, 40,* 216-231.

Costello, J. (1977). Programmed instruction. *Journal of Speech and Hearing Disorders, 42,* 3-28.

Costello, J.M. (1983). Current behavioral treatments for children In D. Prins & R. Ingham (Eds.), *Treatment of stuttering in early childhood: Methods and issues .* San Diego: College-Hill Press.

Costello, J.M. (1984) Operant conditioning and the treatment of stuttering.In W.H. Perkins (Ed.), *Current therapy of communication disorders: Stuttering disorders .* New York: Thieme-Stratton.

Costello, J.M., & Hurst, M. R. (1981). An analysis of the relationship among stuttering behaviors. *Journal of Speech and Hearing Research,, 24,* 247-256.

Costello, J.M., & Ingham, R.J.(1984a). Assessment strategies for stuttering. In R.F. Curlee & W.H. Perkins (Eds.), *Nature and treatment of stuttering: New directions .* San Diego: College-Hill Press.

Costello, J.M., & Ingham, R.J.(1984b). Stuttering as an operant disorder. In R.F. Curlee & W.H. Perkins (Eds.), *Nature and treatment of stuttering: New directions .* San Diego: College-Hill Press.

Cox, N.J., Seider, R.A., & Kidd, K.K. (1984) Some environmental factors and hypotheses for stuttering in families with several stutterers. *Journal of Speech and Hearing Research, 27,* 543-548.

Craig, A. (1989). In defence of smooth speech treatments: A response to Onslow and Ingham's paper "Whither prolonged speech? The disquieting evolution of a stuttering therapy procedure." *Australian Journal of Human Communication, 17,* 61-68.

Craig, A. (1990). An investigation into the relationship between anxiety and stuttering. *Journal of Speech and Hearing Disorders, 55,* 290-294.

Craig, A.R., & Andrews, G. (1985). The prediction and prevention of relapse in stuttering: The value of self-control techniques and locus of control measures. *Behavior Modification, 9,* 427-442.

Craig, A.R., Feyer, A.-M., & Andrews, G. (1987). An overview of a behavioural treatment for stuttering. *Australian Psychologist, 22,* 53-62.

Craig, A.R., Franklin, J. A., & Andrews, G. (1984). A scale to measure locus of control of behaviour. *British Journal of Medical Psychology, 57,* 173-180.

Craig, A.R., & Howie, P.M. (1982). Locus of control and maintenance of behavioural therapy skills. *British Journal of Clinical Psychology, 21,* 65-66.

Cullinan, W., & Prather, E. (1968). Reliability of "live" ratings of the speech of stutterers. *Perceptual and Motor Skills, 27,* 403-409.

Culp, D. (1984). The preschool fluency development program: Assessment and Treatment. In M. Peins (Ed.), *Contemporary approaches in stuttering therapy* . Boston: Little, Brown and Company.

Curlee, R.F. (1980). A case selection strategy for young disfluent children. *Seminars in Speech and Language, 1,* 277-287.

Curlee, R.F. (1981). Observer agreement on disfluency and stuttering. *Journal of Speech and Hearing Research, 24,* 595-600.

Curlee, R.F. (1984). Stuttering disorders: An overview. In J. Costello (Ed.), *Speech disorders in children* . San Diego: College-Hill.

Curlee, R.F. (1993). Identification and management of beginning stuttering. In R. F. Curlee (Ed.). *Stuttering and related disorders of fluency* . New York: Thieme Medical Publishers.

Curlee, R.F., & Perkins, W.H. (1969). Conversational rate control therapy for stuttering. *Journal of Speech and Hearing Disorders, 34,* 245-250.

Curlee, R.F., & Perkins, W.H. (Eds.) (1984). *Nature and treatment of stuttering: New directions* . San Diego: College-Hill Press.

Darley, F.L. (1955). The relationship of parental attitudes and adjustments to the development of stuttering. In W. Johnson & R.R. Leutenegger (Eds.), *Stuttering in children and adults* . Minneapolis: University of Minnesota Press.

DeJoy, D., & Gregory, H. (1985). The relationship between age and frequency of disfluency in preschool children. *Journal of Fluency Disorders, 10,* 107-122.

Dickson, S. (1971). Incipient stuttering and spontaneous remission of stuttered speech. *Journal of Communication Disorders, 4,* 99-110.

DeNil, L.F., & Brutten, G. (1991). Speech-associated attitudes of stuttering and nonstuttering children. *Journal of Speech and Hearing Research, 34,* 60-66.

Di Simoni, F.G. (1974). Some preliminary observations on temporal compensation in the speech of children. *Journal of the Acoustical Society of America, 56,* 697-699.

Eisenson, J. (1958). A perseverative theory of stuttering. In J. Eisenson (Ed.), *Stuttering: A symposium.* New York: Harper and Row.

Erickson, R.L. (1969). Assessing communication attitudes among stutterers. *Journal of Speech and Hearing Research, 12,* 711-724.

Estes, W.K., & Skinner, B.F. (1941). Some quantitative properties of anxiety. *Journal of Experimental Psychology, 21,* 390-400.

Eve, C., Onslow, M., Andrews, C., & Adams, R. (1993). Measuring the severity of early stuttering: The reliability of a 10-point scale. *Manuscript submitted for publication.*

Eysenck, H.J. (1952). The effects of psychotherapy: An evaluation. *Journal of Consulting Psychology, 16,* 319-324.

Fairbanks, G. (1954). Systematic research in experimental phonetics: I. A theory of the speech mechanism as a servosystem. *Journal of Speech and Hearing Disorders, 19,* 133-139.

Farber, S. (1981). *Identical twins reared apart: A reanalysis.* New York: Basic Books.

Faust, D. (1984). *The limits of scientific reasoning.* Minneapolis: University of Minnesota Press.

Few, L.R., & Lingwall, J. (1972). A further analysis of fluency within stuttered speech. *Journal of Speech and Hearing Research, 15,* 356-363.

Finn, P., & Gow, M. (1989). Predictions of outcome after treatment for stuttering. *British Journal of Psychiatry, 154,* 273-274.

Finn, P., & Ingham, R.J. (1989). The selection of "fluent" samples in research on stuttering: Conceptual and methodological considerations. *Journal of Speech and Hearing Research, 32,* 401-418.

Flanagan, B., Goldiamond, I., & Azrin, N. (1958). Operant stuttering: The control of stuttering behavior through response-contingent consequences. *Journal of the Experimental Analysis of Behavior, 1,* 173-178.

Fowler, S.C., & Ingham, R.J. (1986). *Stuttering treatment rating recorder.* Santa Barbara: University of California, Santa Barbara.

Franck, R. (1980). Integration of an intensive program for stutterers within the normal activities of a major acute hospital. *Australian Journal of Human Communication Disorders, 8,* 4-15.

Franken, M.C., Boves, L., Peters, H.F.M., & Webster, R.L. (1992). Perceptual evaluation of the speech before and after fluency shaping stuttering therapy. *Journal of Fluency Disorders, 17,* 223-241.

Franken, M.C., Peters, H.F.M., & Tettero, C.M. (1989). Evaluation of the Dutch adaptation of Webster's Precision Fluency Shaping program for stutterers. Proceedings of the *XXIst Congress of the International Association of Logopedics and Phoniatrics,* Volume 1.

Freeman, F., & Ushijima, T. (1978). Laryngeal muscle activity during stuttering. *Journal of Speech and Hearing Research, 21,* 538-562.

Froeschels, E. (1915). Stuttering and nystagmus. *Monatschrift fur Ohrenheilkunde, 49,* 161-167.

Froeschels, E. (1933). *Speech therapy.* Boston: Expression Co..

Gladstein, K.L., Seider, R.A., & Kidd, K.K. (1981) Analysis of the sibship pattterns of stutterers. *Journal of Speech and Hearing Research, 24*, 460-462.

Glasner, P., & Rosenthal, D. (1957). Parental diagnosis of stuttering in young children. *Journal of Speech and Hearing Disorders, 22*, 288-295.

Goldiamond, I. (1965). Stuttering and fluency as manipulatable operant response classes. In L. Krasner & L.P. Ullman (Eds.), *Research in behavior modification.* New York: Holt, Rinehart & Winston.

Gregory, H. (1984). *Prevention of stuttering: Management of early stages.* San Diego: College-Hill Press.

Gregory, H. (1986). Stuttering: Differential Evaluation and Therapy. Austin: Pro-Ed.

Gregory, H.H., & Hill, D. (1980). Stuttering therapy for children. *Seminars in Speech and Language, 1,* 351-363.

Guitar, B. (1976). Pretreatment factors associated with the outcome of stuttering therapy. *Journal of Speech and Hearing Research, 19,* 590-600.

Guitar, B. (1979). A response to Ingham's critique. *Journal of Speech and Hearing Disorders, 44,* 400-403.

Guitar, B., & Bass, C. (1978). Stuttering therapy: The relation between attitude change and long-term outcome. *Journal of Speech and Hearing Disorders, 43,* 392-400.

Guitar, B., Schaefer, H.K., Donahue-Kilburg, G., & Bond, L. (1992). Parent verbal interactions and speech rate: A case study in stuttering. *Journal of Speech and Hearing Research, 35(4),* 742-754.

Hall, D.H., & Yairi, E. (1992). Fundamental frequency, jitter, and shimmer in preschoolers who stutter. *Journal of Speech and Hearing Research, 35,* 1002-1008.

Ham, R.E. (1989). What are we measuring? *Journal of Fluency Disorders, 14,* 231-243.

Hamre, C. (1992). Stuttering prevention I: Primacy of identification. *Journal of Fluency Disorders, 17,* 3-23.

Healey, E.C., & Gutkin, B. (1984). Analysis of stutterers voice onset times and fundamental frequency contours during fluency. *Journal of Speech and Hearing Research, 27,* 219-225.

Healey, E.C., & Ramig, P.R. (1986). Acoustic measures of stutterers' and nonstutterers' fluency in two speech contexts. *Journal of Speech and Hearing Research, 29,* 325-331.

Helm-Estabrooks, N. (1993). Stuttering associated with acquired neurological disorders. In R. F. Curlee (Ed.), *Stuttering and related disorders of fluency* . Thieme Medical Publishers: New York.

Hillman, R.E., & Gilbert, H.R. (1977). Voice onset time for voiceless stop consonants in the fluent reading of stutterers and nonstutterers. *Journal of the Acoustical Society of America, 61,* 610-611.

Horii, Y., & Ramig, P.R. (1987). Pause and utterance durations and fundamental frequency characteristics of repeated oral readings by stutterers and nonstutterers. *Journal of Fluency Disorders, 12,* 257-270.

Howie, P.M. (1981). Concordance for stuttering in monozygotic and dizygotic twin pairs. *Journal of Speech and Hearing Research, 24,* 317-321.

Howie, P., & Andrews, G. (1984). Treatment of adults: Managing fluency. In R.F. Curlee and W.H. Perkins (Eds.) *Nature and treatment of stuttering: New directions* . San Diego: College-Hill Press.

Howie, P., Andrews, G., & Tanner, S. (1978). An intensive behaviour modification programme for the treatment of stutterers. *Australian Behaviour Therapist, 5,* 17-19.

Howie, P.M., Tanner, S., & Andrews, G. (1981). Short- and long-term outcome in an intensive treatment program for adult stutterers. *Journal of Speech and Hearing Disorders, 46,* 104-109.

Hubbard, C.P., & Yairi, E. (1988). Clustering of disfluencies in the speech of stuttering and nonstuttering preschool children. *Journal of Speech and Hearing Research, 31,* 228-233.

Ingham, J.C. (1993). Behavioral treatment of stuttering children. In R. F. Curlee (Ed.), *Stuttering and related disorders of fluency* . New York: Thieme Medical Publishers.

Ingham, J.C. (in press). Therapy of the stuttering child. In G. Blanken, J. Dittman, H. Grimm, J.C. Marshall, C.-W. Wallesch (Eds.), *Linguistic Disorders and pathologies.* Berlin: Walter De Gruyter.

Ingham, J.C, & Ingham, R.J. (1987). *Stuttering measurement training.* Santa Barbara: University of California, Santa Barbara.

Ingham, R.J. (1976). "Onset, prevalence, and recovery from stuttering": A reassessment of findings from the Andrews and Harris study. *Journal of Speech and Hearing Disorders, 41,* 280-281.

Ingham, R.J. (1977). Towards an accountability model for the management of stuttering. Paper read to the *Victorian Department of Education Speech Therapists' In-Service Training Meeting,* Melbourne, May.

Ingham, R.J. (1979). Comment on "Stuttering therarpy: The relation between attitude change and long-term outcome." *Journal of Speech and Hearing Disorders, 44,* 397-400.

Ingham, R.J. (1980). Modification of maintenance and generalization during stuttering treatment. *Journal of Speech and Hearing Research, 23,* 732-745.

Ingham, R.J. (1981a). Evaluation and maintenance in stuttering treatment: A search for ecstasy with nothing but agony. In E. Boberg (Ed.), *Maintenance of fluency*. New York: Elsevier.

Ingham, R.J. (1981b). *Stuttering therapy manual: Hierarchy control schedule*. Sydney: Australia. Cumberland College Press.

Ingham, R.J. (1982). The effects of self-evaluation training on maintenance and generalization during stuttering treatment. *Journal of Speech and Hearing Disorders, 47*, 271-280.

Ingham, R.J. (1983) Stuttering and spontaneous remission: When will the emperor realize he has no clothes on? In D. Prins & R.J. Ingham (Eds.), *Treatment of stuttering in early childhood: Methods and issues* . San Diego: College-Hill Press.

Ingham, R.J. (1984). *Stuttering and behavior therapy: Current status and experimental foundations*. San Diego: College-Hill Press.

Ingham, R.J. (1987). *Residential prolonged speech stuttering therapy manual*. Santa Barbara: Department of Speech and Hearing Sciences, University of California.

Ingham, R.J. (1990a). Commentary on Perkins (1990) and Moore and Perkins (1990): On the valid role of reliability in identifying "what is stuttering." *Journal of Speech and Hearing Disorders, 55*, 394-397.

Ingham, R.J. (1990b). Stuttering. In A. S. Bellack, M. Hersen, & A.E. Kazdin (Eds.), *International handbook of behavior modification and therapy* (2nd. Ed.). Plenum Press: New York.

Ingham, R. (1990c). *Stuttering: recent trends in research and therapy*. In H. Winitz (Ed.), *Human communication and its disorders*. Norwood, NJ: Ablex.

Ingham, R.J. (in preparation). *Stuttering and behavior therapy: Current status and experimental foundations* (2nd. Ed.).

Ingham, R.J., & Andrews, G. (1973). Details of a token economy stuttering therapy programme for adults. *Australian Journal of Human Communication Disorders, 1*, 13-20.

Ingham, R.J. & Cordes, A.K. (1992). Interclinic differences in stuttering-event counts. *Journal of Fluency Disorders, 17*, 171-176.

Ingham, R.J., Cordes, A.K., & Gow, M.L. (1992). Time-interval measurement of stuttering: Modifying interjudge agreement. *Journal of Speech and Hearing Research, 36*, 503-515.

Ingham, R.J., Gow, M., & Costello, J.M. (1985). Stuttering and speech naturalness: Some additional data.*Journal of Speech and Hearing Disorders, 50*, 217-219.

Ingham, R.J., Ingham, J.C., Onslow, M., & Finn, P. (1989). Stutterers' self-ratings of speech naturalness: Assessing effects and reliability. *Journal of Speech and Hearing Research, 32*, 419-431.

Ingham, R.J., Martin, R.R., Haroldson, S.K., Onslow, M., & Leney, M. (1985) Modification of listener-judged naturalness in the speech of stutterers. *Journal of Speech and Hearing Research, 28*, 495-504.

Ingham, R.J., Montgomery, G., & Ulliana, L.(1983). The effect of manipulating phonation duration on stuttering. *Journal of Speech and Hearing Research, 26*, 579-587.

Ingham, R.J., & Onslow, M. (1983) *Stuttering Treatment Evaluation Manual*. Sydney: Cumberland College of Health Sciences.

Ingham, R.J. & Onslow, M. (1985). Measurement and modification of speech naturalness during stuttering therapy. *Journal of Speech and Hearing Disorders, 50*, 261-281.

Ingham, R.J. & Onslow, M. (1987). Generalization and maintenance of treatment benefits for children who stutter. *Seminars in Speech and Language, 8*, 303-326.

Ingham, R.J. & Onslow, M. (1990). More on "Whither prolonged speech": A response to Craig (1989). *Australian Journal of Human Communication Disorders, 18*, 102-105.

Ingham, R.J., & Packman, A. (1977). Treatment and generalization effects in an experimental treatment for a stutterer using contingency management and speech rate control. *Journal of Speech and Hearing Disorders, 42*, 394-407.

Ingham, R.J., Southwood, H., & Horsburgh, G. (1981). Some effects of the Edinburgh Masker on stuttering during oral reading and spontaneous speech. *Journal of Fluency Disorders, 6*, 135-154.

Irwin, A. (1988). *Stammering in young children: A practical self-help programme for parents*. Northhamptonshire: Thorsons Publishing Group.

James, J.E. (1976). The influence of duration on the effects of time-out from speaking.*Journal of Speech and Hearing Research , 19*, 206-215

James, J.E. (1981a). Self-monitoring of stuttering: Reactivity and accuracy. *Behavior Research and Therapy, 19*, 291-296.

James, J.E. (1981b). Behavioral self-control of stuttering using time-out from speaking. *Journal of Applied Behavior Analysis, 14*, 25-37.

James, J.E. (1981c). Punishment of stuttering: Contingency and stimulus parameters. *Journal of Communication Disorders, 14*, 375-386.

James, J.E. (1983). Parameters of the influence of self-initiated time-out from speaking on stuttering. *Journal of Communication Disorders, 16*, 123-132.

James, J., Ricciardelli, L., Hunter, C., & Rogers, P. (1989). Relative efficacy of intensive and spaced behavioral treatment of stuttering. *Behavior Modification, 13,* 376-395.

Johnson, G.F., Coleman, K., & Rasmussen, K. (1978). Multidays: Multidimensional approach for the young stutterer. *Language, Speech and Hearing Services in Schools, 9,* 129-132.

Johnson, J.M., & Pennypacker, H.S. (1980). *Strategies and tactics of human behavioral research.* Hillsdale, NJ: Lawrence Erlbaum Associates.

Johnson, L. (1984). Facilitating parental involvement in therapy of the preschool disfluent child. In W. H. Perkins (Ed.), *Stuttering disorders.* New York: Thieme-Stratton.

Johnson, L.H. (1980). Facilitating parental involvement in therapy of the disfluent child. *Seminars in Speech and Language, 1,* 301-309.

Johnson, W. (1942). A study of the onset and development of stuttering. *Journal of Speech and Hearing Disorders, 7,* 251-257.

Johnson, W. (1955). The time, the place, and the problem. In W. Johnson & R.R. Leutenegger (Eds.). *Stuttering in Children and Adults.* Minneapolis: University of Minnesota Press.

Johnson, W. (1967). An open letter to the mother of a stuttering child. In W. Johnson and D. Moeller (Eds.), *Speech handicapped school children* (3rd Ed.). New York: Harper and Row.

Johnson, W., & Associates (1959). *The onset of stuttering.* Minneapolis: University of Minneapolis Press.

Johnson, W., Darley, F.L., & Spriestersbach, D.C. (1963). *Diagnostic methods in speech pathology.* New York: Harper and Row.

Johnson, W. & Leutenegger, R.R. (Eds.) (1955). *Stuttering in children and adults .* Minneapolis: University of Minnesota Press.

Jones, R.J., & Azrin, N.H. (1969). Behavioral engineering: Stuttering as a function of stimulus duration during speech synchronization. *Journal of Applied Behavior Analysis, 2,* 223-229.

Kazdin, A.E. (1978). Behavior therapy: Evolution and expansion. *The Counseling Psychologist, 7,* 34-37.

Kelly, E.M., & Conture, E.G. (1992). Speaking rates, response time latencies, and interrupting behaviors of young stutterers, nonstutterers, and their mothers. *Journal of Speech and Hearing Research, 35,* 1256-1267.

Kidd, K.K. (1977). A genetic perspective on stuttering. *Journal of Fluency Disorders, 2,* 259-269.

Kidd, K.K. (1980). Genetic models of stuttering. *Journal of Fluency Disorders, 5,* 187-201.

Kidd, K.K. (1984). Stuttering as a genetic disorder. In R.F. Curlee and W.H. Perkins (Eds.), *Nature and treatment of stuttering: New directions .* San Diego: College-Hill Press.

Kirschenbaum, D., & Tomarken, A. (1982). *On facing the generalization problem: The study of self-regulatory failure.* New York: Academic Press.

Koegel, R.L., Koegel, L.K., Van Voy, K., & Ingham, J.C. (1989). Within-clinic versus outside-of-clinic self-monitoring of articulation to promote generalization. *Journal of Speech and Hearing Disorders, 53,* 392-399.

Kowal, S., O'Connell, D.C, & Sabin, E.F. (1975). Development of temporal patterning and vocal hesitations in spontaneous narratives. *Journal of Psycholinguistic Research, 4,* 195-207.

Kraaimaat, F., Janssen, P., & Brutten, G. (1988). The relationship between stutterers' cognitive and autonomic anxiety and therapy outcome. *Journal of Fluency Disorders, 13,* 107-113.

Kraaimaat, F., Janssen, P., & Van Dam-Baggen, R. (1991). Social anxiety and stuttering. *Perceptual and Motor Skills, 72,* 766.

Krikorian, C., & Runyan, C. (1983). A perceptual comparison: Stuttering and nonstuttering children's nonstuttered speech. *Journal of Fluency Disorders, 8,* 283-290.

Kroll, R., & O'Keefe, B. (1985). Molecular self-analyses of stuttered speech via speech time expansion . *Journal of Fluency Disorders, 10,* 93-105.

Kully, D., & Boberg, E. (1988). An investigation of interclinic agreement in the identification of fluent and stuttered syllables. *Journal of Fluency Disorders, 13,* 309-318.

La Croix, Z.E. (1972). Management of disfluent speech through self-monitoring procedures. *Journal of Speech and Hearing Disorders, 38,* 272-274.

La Point, L.L., & Horner, J. (1981). Palilalia: A descriptive study of pathological reiterative utterances. *Journal of Speech and Hearing Disorders, 46,* 34-38.

Lankford, S., & Cooper, E. (1974). Recovery from stuttering as viewed by parents of self-diagnosed recovered stutterers. *Journal of Communication Disorders, 7,* 171-180.

Lass, N.J., Ruscello, D.M., Pannbacker, M.D., Schmitt, J.F., & Everly-Myers, D. S. (1989). Speech-language pathologists' perceptions of child and adult female and male stutterers. *Journal of Fluency Disorders, 14,* 127-134.

Leach, E. (1969). Stuttering: Clinical application of response-contingent procedures. In B.B. Gray & G. England (Eds.), *Stuttering and the conditioning therapies.* California: Monterey Institute of Speech and Hearing.

Leith, W., & Timmons, J. (1983). The stutterer's reaction to the telephone as a speaking situation. *Journal of Fluency Disorders, 8*, 233-243.

Lemert, E. (1953). Some Indians who stutter. *Journal of Speech and Hearing Disorders, 18*, 168-174.

Lewis, B. A. (1990). Familial phonological disorders: Four pedigrees. *Journal of Speech and Hearing Disorders, 55*, 160-170.

Lincoln, M., and Onslow, M. (1992). The role of anxiety in stuttering: Implications for treatment. Paper presented at the *Annual Conference of the Australian Association of Speech and Hearing, Melbourne*, February.

Love, L.R., & Jeffress, L.A. (1971). Identification of brief pauses in the fluent speech of stutterers and nonstutterers. *Journal of Speech and Hearing Research, 14*, 229-240.

Luper, H., & Mulder, R. (1964). *Stuttering: Therapy for children*. Englewood Cliffs, New Jersey: Prentice-Hall.

MacKay, D.G. & MacDonald, M.C. (1984) Stuttering as a sequencing and timing disorder. In R.F. Curlee & W. H. Perkins (Eds.) *Nature and treatment of stuttering: New directions*. San Diego: College-Hill Press.

Mahr, G., & Leith, W. (1992). Psychogenic stuttering of adult onset. *Journal of Speech and Hearing Research, 35*, 283-286.

Mallard, A.R., Gardner, L.S., & Downey, C.S. (1988). Clinical training in stuttering for school clinicians. *Journal of Fluency Disorders, 13*, 253-259.

Mallard, A., & Kelley, J. (1982). The Precision Fluency Shaping Program: Replication and evaluation. *Journal of Fluency Disorders, 7*, 287-294.

Mallard, A.R., & Westbrook, J.B. (1985). Vowel duration in stutterers participating in precision fluency shaping. *Journal of Fluency Disorders, 10*, 221-228.

Manning, W., Trutna, P., & Shaw, C. (1976). Verbal versus tangible reward for children who stutter. *Journal of Speech and Hearing Disorders, 41*, 52-62.

Manusu, R., Boycott, N., Grant, S., & Khanbhai, F. (1992). *Speech Pathology Department patient manual: Stuttering treatment programme*. Sydney: Royal Prince Alfred Hospital.

Martin, M., & Kinnear, J. (1985) *Genetics: A human focus*. Melbourne: Nelson.

Martin, R.R. (1981) Introduction and perspective: Review of published research. In E. Boberg (Ed.), *Maintenance of fluency*. New York: Elsevier.

Martin, R.R., & Berndt, L.A. (1970). The effects of time-out on stuttering in a 12-year-old boy. *Exceptional Children, 36*, 303-304.

Martin, R.R, & Haroldson, S.K. (1981). Stuttering identification: Standard definition and moment of stuttering. *Journal of Speech and Hearing Research, 46*, 59-63.

Martin, R.R., & Haroldson, S.K. (1982). Contingent self stimulation for stuttering. *Journal of Speech and Hearing Disorders, 47*, 407-413.

Martin, R.R. & Haroldson, S.K. (1986). Stuttering as involuntary loss of speech control: Barking up a new tree. *Journal of Speech and Hearing Disorders, 51*, 187-190.

Martin, R.R., & Haroldson, S.K. (1992). Stuttering and speech naturalness: Audio and audiovisual judgments. *Journal of Speech and Hearing Research, 35*, 521-528.

Martin, R.R., Haroldson, S.K.,'& Triden, K.A. (1984). Stuttering and speech naturalness. *Journal of Speech and Hearing Disorders, 49*, 53-58.

Martin, R.R., Kuhl, P., & Haroldson, S. (1972) An experimental treatment with two preschool stuttering children. *Journal of Speech and Hearing Research, 15*, 743-752.

Martin, R.R., & Lindamood, L.P. (1986). Stuttering and spontaneous recovery: Implications for the speech-language pathologist. *Language, Speech, and Hearing Services in Schools, 17*, 207-218.

Martin, R.R., & Siegel, G.M. (1966a). The effects of response contingent shock on stuttering. *Journal of Speech and Hearing Research, 9*, 340-352..

Martin, R.R., & Siegel, G.M. (1966b). The effects of simultaneously punishing stuttering and rewarding fluency. *Journal of Speech and Hearing Research, 9*, 466-475.

Martyn, M.M., & Sheehan, J. (1968). Onset of stuttering and recovery. *Behaviour Research and Therapy, 6*, 295-307.

McClean, M.D. (1990). Neuromotor aspects of stuttering: Levels of impairment and disability. *ASHA Reports, 18*, 64-71.

McDermott, L.D. (1971). Clinical management of stuttering behavior: A case study. *Feedback, 1*, 6-7.

McGarr, M.S. (1983). The intelligibility of deaf speech to experienced and inexperienced listeners. *Journal of Speech and Hearing Research, 26*, 3, 451-458.

Metz, D.E., Conture, E.G., & Caruso, A. (1979). Voice onset time, frication, and aspiration during stutterers' fluent speech. *Journal of Speech and Hearing Research, 22*, 649-656.

Metz, D.E., Onufrak, J.A., & Ogburn, R.S. (1979). An acoustical analysis of stutterer's speech prior to and at the termination of speech therapy. *Journal of Fluency Disorders, 4,* 249-254.

Metz, D.E., Samar, V.J., & Sacco, P.R. (1983). Acoustic analysis of stutterers' fluent speech before and after therapy. *Journal of Speech and Hearing Research, 26,* 531-536.

Metz, D.E., Schiavetti, N., & Sacco, P.R. (1990). Acoustic and psychophysical dimensions of the perceived speech naturalness of nonstutterers and posttreatment stutterers. *Journal of Speech and Hearing Disorders, 55,* 516-525.

Meyers, S.C. (1989). Nonfluencies of preschool stutterers and conversational partners: Observing reciprocal relationships. *Journal of Speech and Hearing Disorders, 54,* 106-112.

Meyers, S.C., & Freeman, F. (1985a). Interruptions as a variable in stuttering and disfluency. *Journal of Speech and Hearing Research, 28,* 428-435.

Meyers, S.C., & Freeman, F. (1985b). Mother and child speech rates as a variable in stuttering and disfluency. *Journal of Speech and Hearing Research, 28,* 436-444.

Miller, N.E. (1944). Experimental studies of conflict. In J. McV. Hunt (Ed.), *Personality and the Behaviour Disorders.* New York: Ronald Press.

Miller, S., & Watson, B. (1992). The relationship between communication attitutde, anxiety and depression in stutterers and nonstutterers. *Journal of Speech and Hearing Research, 35,* 789-798.

Mooney, J. (1990). Stutterers master smooth speech. *Australian Doctor Weekly, 26-27,* June.

Moore, S.E., & Perkins, W.H. (1990). Validity and reliability of judgements of authentic and simulated stuttering. *Journal of Speech and Hearing Disorders, 55,* 383-391.

Moore, W.H. (1984). Central nervous system characteristics of stutterers. In R.F. Curlee & W.H. Perkins (Eds.), *Nature and Treatment of stuttering: New directions.* San Diego: College-Hill Press.

Moore, W.H. (1986). Hemispheric alpha asymmetries of stutterers and non-stutterers for the recall and recognition of words and connected reading passages: Some relationships to severity of stuttering. *Journal of Fluency Disorders, 11,* 71-89.

Moore, W.H. (1990). Pathophysiology of stuttering: Cerebral activation differences in stutterers. *ASHA Reports, 18,* 72-80.

Moore, W.H., & Haynes, W.C. (1980). Alpha hemispheric asymmetry and stuttering: Some support from a segmentation dysfunction hypothesis. *Journal of Speech and Hearing Research, 23,* 229-247.

Morris-Yates, A., Andrews, G., Howie, P., & Henderson, A. (1990). Twins: A test of the equal environments assumption. *Acta Psychiatrica Scandinavia, 81,* 322-326.

Mowrer, D.E. (1975). An instructional program to increase fluent speech of stutterers. *Journal of Fluency Disorders, 1,* 25-35.

Mower, D.E. (1982). *Methods of modifying speech behaviors* (2nd Ed.). Columbus, OH: Charles E. Merrill.

Mowrer, D.E. (1987). Repetition of final consonants in the speech of a young child. *Journal of Speech and Hearing Disorders, 52,* 174-178.

Mysak, E. (1960). Servo-theory and stuttering. *Journal of Speech and Hearing Disorders, 25,* 188-195.

Neilson, M., & Andrews, G. (1993). Intensive fluency training of chronic stutterers. In R. F. Curlee (Ed.), *Stuttering and related disorders of fluency .* New York: Thieme Medical Publishers.

Neilson, M.D., & Neilson, P.D. (1987). Speech motor control and stuttering: A computational model of adaptive sensory-motor processing. *Speech Communication, 6,* 325-333.

Netsell, R. (1986). *A neurological view of speech production and the dysarthrias.* San Diego: College-Hill.

Nittrouer, S., & Cheney, C. (1984). Operant techniques used in stuttering therapy: A review. *Journal of Fluency Disorders, 9,* 169-190.

O'Keefe, B., & Kroll, R. (1980). Clinician's molar and molecular stuttering analyses of expanded and nonexpanded speech. *Journal of Fluency Disorders, 5,* 43-54.

Onslow, M. (1992a). Identification of early stuttering: Issues and suggested strategies. *American Journal of Speech-Language Pathology, 1,* 21-27.

Onslow, M. (1992b). Choosing a treatment procedure for early stuttering: Issues and future directions. *Journal of Speech and Hearing Research, 35,* 983-993.

Onslow, M., Adams, R., & Ingham, R. (1991) Reliability of speech naturalness ratings of stuttered speech during treatment. *Journal of Speech and Hearing Research, 35,* 994-1001.

Onslow, M., Andrews, C., & Costa, L. (1990). Parental Severity Scaling of Early Stuttered Speech: Four Case Studies. *Australian Journal of Human Communication Disorders, 18,* 47-61.

Onslow, M., Andrews, C., & Lincoln, M. (in press). A control/experimental trial of an operant treatment for early stuttering. *Journal of Speech and Hearing Research..*

Onslow, M. & Costa, L. (1989). When the tail begins to wag the dog: Some views on the relationship between speech pathologists and self-help groups in the management of stuttering. *Australian Journal of Human Communication Disorders, 17,* 77-86.

Onslow, M., Costa, L., & Rue, S. (1990). Direct early intervention with stuttering: Some preliminary data. *Journal of Speech and Hearing Disorders, 55,* 405-416.

Onslow, M., Gardner, K.M., Bryant, K., Stuckings, C.L., & Knight, T. (1992). Stuttered and normal speech events in early childhood: The validity of a behavioral data language. *Journal of Speech and Hearing Research, 35,* 79-87.

Onslow, M., Harrison, E., & Jones, A. (1993). Early stuttering: Onset, treatment, and recovery. Paper presented at the *Annual Conference of the Australian Association of Speech and Hearing,* Darwin, May.

Onslow, M., Hayes, B., Hutchins, L., & Newman, D. (1992). Speech naturalness and prolonged-speech treatments for stuttering: Further variables and data. *Journal of Speech and Hearing Research, 35,* 274-282.

Onslow, M., & Ingham, R.J. (1987). Speech quality measurement and the management of stuttering. *Journal of Speech and Hearing Disorders, 52,* 2-17.

Onslow, M., & Ingham, R.J. (1989). Whither prolonged speech? The disquieting evolution of a stuttering therapy procedure. *Australian Journal of Human Communication Disorders, 17,* 67-81.

Onslow, M., van Doorn, J., & Newman, D. (1992). Variability of acoustic segment durations after prolonged-speech treatment for stuttering. *Journal of Speech and Hearing Research, 35,* 529-536.

Orton, S. (1927). Studies in stuttering. *Archives of Neurology and Psychiatry, 18,* 671-672.

Packman, A., Ingham, R.J. & Onslow, M. (1993). Reliability of listeners' stuttering counts: The effect of instructions designed to reduce ambiguity. *Manuscript submitted for publication.*

Packman, A., Onslow, M., & van Doorn, J. (in press). Prolonged speech and the modification of stuttering: Perceptual, acoustic, and electroglottographic data. *Journal of Speech and Hearing Research.*

Packman, A., Van Doorn, J., & Onslow, M. (1992). Stuttering treatments: What is happening to the acoustic signal? In J. Pittam (Ed.) *Proceedings of the Fourth Australian International Conference on Speech Science and Technology.* Brisbane, December.

Pauls, D.L. (1990). A review of the evidence for genetic factors in stuttering. *ASHA Reports, 18,* 34-38.

Perkins, W.H. (1983a). The problem of definition: Commentary on "stuttering". *Journal of Speech and Hearing Disorders, 48,* 226-246.

Perkins, W.H. (1983b). Onset of stuttering: The case of the missing block. In D. Prins & R.J. Ingham (Eds.), *Treatment of stuttering in early childhood: Methods and issues.*San Diego: College-Hill Press.

Perkins, W.H. (1984). Stuttering as a categorical event: Barking up the wrong tree. *Journal of Speech and Hearing Disorders, 49,* 431-434.

Perkins, W.H. (1986). More bite for a bark: Epilogue to Martin and Haroldson's letter. *Journal of Speech and Hearing Disorders, 51,* 190-191.

Perkins, W.H. (1990a). What is stuttering? *Journal of Speech and Hearing Disorders, 55,* 370-382.

Perkins, W. (1990b). Gratitude, good intentions, and red herrings: A response to commentaries. *Journal of Speech and Hearing Disorders , 55,* 402-404.

Perkins, W.H. (1992). *Stuttering prevented.* San Diego: Singular Publishing Group.

Peters, A. D. (1977). The effect of positive reinforcement on fluency: Two case studies. *Language, Speech and Hearing Services in Schools, 8,*15-22.

Peters, F.M., & Hulstijn, W.(Eds.) (1987).*Speech motor dynamics and stuttering.* New York: Springer-Verlag.

Peters, F.M., & Hulstijn, W., & Starkweather, C.W. (Eds.) (1987).*Speech motor control and stuttering.* Amsterdam: Elsevier.

Peters, T.J., and Guitar, B. (1991) *Stuttering: An integrated approach to its treatment.* Baltimore: Williams and Wilkins.

Pindzola, R.H. (1987). Durational characteristics of the fluent speech of stutterers and nonstutterers. *Folia Phoniatrica, 39,* 90-97.

Pindzola, R.K., & White, D.T. (1986). A protocol for differentiating the incipient stutterer. *Language, Speech and Hearing Services in Schools, 17,* 2-15.

Postma, A., & Kolk, H. (1992). Error monitoring in people who stutter: Evidence against auditory feedback defect theories. *Journal of Speech and Hearing Research, 35,* 1024-1032.

Poulos, M., & Webster, W. (1991). Family history as a basis for subgrouping people who stutter. *Journal of Speech and Hearing Research, 34,* 5-10.

Prins, D. (1983). Continuity, fragmentation, and tension: Hypotheses applied to evaluation and intervention with preschool disfluent children. In D. Prins & R.J. Ingham (Eds.),*Treatment of stuttering in early childhood: Methods and issues.*San Diego: College-Hill Press.

Prins, D. (1993). Management of stuttering: Treatment of adolescents and adults. In R. F. Curlee (Ed.),*Stuttering and related disorders of fluency .* New York: Thieme Medical Publishers.

Prins, D., & Hubbard, C.P. (1988). Response contingent stimuli and stuttering: Issues and implications.*Journal of Speech and Hearing Research, 31*, 696-709.

Prins, D., & Ingham, R.J. (Eds.) (1983). *Treatment of stuttering in early childhood: Methods and Issues.* San Diego: College-Hill Press.

Prins, D., & Ingham, R.J. (1983). Issues and perspectives. In D. Prins & R. Ingham (Eds.). *Treatment of stuttering in early childhood: Methods and Issues.* San Diego: College-Hill Press.

Ramig, P.R. (1984). Rate changes in the speech of stutterers after therapy. *Journal of Fluency Disorders, 9*, 285-294.

Ramig, P.R. (1993). High reported spontaneous stuttering recovery rates: Fact or fiction? *Language, Speech, and Hearing Services in Schools, 24*, 156-160.

Ratner, N.B. (1992). Measurable outcomes of instructions to modify normal parent-child verbal interactions: Implications for ¬direct stuttering therapy. *Journal of Speech and Hearing Research, 35*, 14-20.

Reed, C.G., & Godden, A.L. (1977). An experimental treatment using verbal punishment with two preschool stutterers. *Journal of Fluency Disorders, 2*, 225-233.

Reed, C.G., & Lingwall, J. (1980). Conditioned stimulus effects on stuttering and GSR's. *Journal of Speech and Hearing Research, 23*, 336-343.

Rickard, H., & Mundy, M. (1965). Direct manipulation of stuttering behavior: An experimental clinical approach. In L.P. Ullmann & L. Krasner (Eds), *Case studies in behavior modification.* New York: Holt, Rinehart and Winston.

Riley, G. (1972). A stuttering severity instrument for children and adults. *Journal of Speech and Hearing Disorders, 37*, 314-322.

Riley, G. (1981). *Stuttering Prediction Instrument.* Tigard, OR: C.C. Publications.

Riley, G.D., & Riley, J. (1983) Evaluation as a basis for intervention. In D. Prins & R. J. Ingham (Eds.), *Treatment of stuttering in early childhood: Methods and issues.* San Diego: College-Hill Press.

Robb, M. P., Lybolt, J. F., & Price, H. A. (1985). Acoustic measures of stutterers' speech following an intensive therapy program. *Journal of Fluency Disorders, 10*, 269-279.

Rosenbek, J.C. (1984). Stuttering secondary to nervous system damage. In R. F. Curlee and W. H. Perkins (Eds.) *Nature and treatment of stuttering: New directions* (31-48). San Diego: College-Hill Press.

Rosenfield, D., & Jerger, J. (1984) Stuttering and auditory function. In R.F. Curlee & W.H. Perkins (Eds.) *Nature and treatment of stuttering: New directions.* San Diego: College-Hill Press.

Rosenfield, D.B., & Nudelman, H.B. (1987). Neuropsychological models of speech dysfluency. In L. Rustin, H. Purser, & D. Rowley (Eds.), *Progress in the treatment of fluency disorders.* London: Taylor & Francis.

Roth, C.R., Aronson, A.E., & Davis, L.J. (1989). Clinical studies in psychogenic stuttering of adult onset. *Journal of Speech and Hearing Disorders, 54*, 634-646.

Rotter, J.B. (1966). Generalized expectancies for internal versus external control of reinforcement. *Psychological Monographs, 80*, 1-20.

Rudmin, F. (1984). Parent's report of stress and articulation oscillation as factors in a preschooler's dysfluencies. *Journal of Fluency Disorders, 9*, 85-87.

Runyan, C.M., Bell, J. N. & Prosek, R.A. (1990). Speech naturalness ratings of treated stutterers. *Journal of Speech and Hearing Disorders, 55*, 434-438.

Runyan, C.M, & Runyan, S.E. (1993). Therapy for school-age stutterers: An update on the fluency rules program. In R. F. Curlee (Ed.). *Stuttering and related disorders of fluency .* New York: Thieme Medical Publishers.

Rustin, L. (1987). The treatment of childhood dysfluency through active parental involvement. In L. Rustin, H. Purser, & D. Rowley (Eds.) *Progress in the treatment of fluency disorders.* London: Taylor & Francis.

Ryan, B.P. (1970). An illustration of operant conditioning therapy for stuttering. In Speech Foundation of America, Publication No.7, *Conditioning in stuttering therapy.* Memphis: Speech Foundation of America.

Ryan, B.P. (1971). Operant procedures applied to stuttering therapy for children. *Journal of Speech and Hearing Disorders, 36*, 264-280.

Ryan, B.P. (1974). *Programmed therapy for stuttering in children and adults.* Springfield, IL: Charles C. Thomas.

Ryan, B.P. (1981). Maintenance programs in progress II. In E. Boberg (Ed.), *Maintenance of Fluency.* New York: Elsevier.

Ryan, B.P., & Van Kirk Ryan, B. (1983). Programmed stuttering therapy for children: Comparison of four establishment programs. *Journal of Fluency Disorders, 8*, 291-321.

Salend, S., & Andress, M. (1984). Decreasing stuttering in an elementary-level student. *Language, Speech and Hearing Services in Schools, 15*, 16-21.

Schwartz, H., & Conture, E. (1988). Subgrouping young stutterers: Preliminary behavioral observations. *Journal of Speech and Hearing Research, 31*, 62-71.

Schwartz, H., Zebrowski, P., & Conture, E. (1990). Behaviors at the onset of stuttering. *Journal of Fluency Disorders, 15*, 77-86.

Schwartz, M. (1974). The core of the stuttering block. *Journal of Speech and Hearing Disorders, 39*, 169-177.

Schwartz, M. (1976). *Stuttering solved.* New York: McGraw-Hill.

Shames, G., & Florance, C. (1980). *Stutter-free speech: A goal for therapy.* Columbus: Charles E. Merrill.

Shames, G.H., & Sherrick, C.E. (1963). A discussion of nonfluency and stuttering as operant behavior. *Journal of Speech and Hearing Disorders, 28*, 3-18.

Shaw, C., & Shrum, W. (1972) The effects of response-contingent reward on the connected speech of children who stutter. *Journal of Speech and Hearing Disorders, 37*, 75-88.

Sheehan, J.G. (1975). Conflict theory and avoidance-reduction therapy. In J. Eisenson (Ed.), *Stuttering: A second symposium.* New York: Harper and Row.

Sheehan, J.G, & Martyn, M.M. (1966). Spontaneous recovery from stuttering. *Journal of Speech and Hearing Research, 9*, 121-135.

Sheehan, J.G., & Martyn, M.M. (1970). Stuttering and its disappearance. *Journal of Speech and Hearing Research, 13*, 279-289.

Sheehan, J.G., & Sheehan, V.M. (1984) Avoidance-reduction therapy: A response-suppression hypothesis. In W.H. Perkins (Ed.), *Current therapy of communication disorders: Stuttering disorders.* New York: Thieme-Stratton.

Shenker, C.R., & Finn, P. (1985). An evaluation of the effects of supplemental "fluency" training during maintenance. *Journal of Fluency Disorders, 10*, 257-267.

Shine, R.E. (1984a). Assessment and fluency training with the young stutterer. In M. Peins (Ed.), *Contemporary approaches in stuttering therapy.* Boston: Little, Brown and Company.

Shine, R.E. (1984b). Direct management of the beginning stutterer. In W. H. Perkins (Ed.), *Stuttering disorders* . New York: Thieme-Stratton.

Sidman, M. (1960). *Tactics of scientific research.* New York: Basic Books.

Siegel, G.M. (1989). Exercises in behavioral explanation. *Journal of Speech-Language Pathology and Audiology, 13*, 3-6.

Siegel, G.M. (1987) The limits of science in communication disorders. *Journal of Speech and Hearing Disorders, 52*, 306-312.

Siegel, G.M. (1990). Concluding remarks. In L.B. Olswang, C.K. Thompson, S. Warren, & N.J. Minghetti, (Eds.), *Treatment efficacy research in communication disorders.* Rockville, MD: American Speech-Language-Hearing Foundation .

Siegel, G.M., & Ingham, R.J. (1987). Theory and science in communciation disorders. *Journal of Speech and Hearing Disorders, 52*, 99-104.

Silverman, E.-M. (1972). Generality of disfluency data collected from preschoolers. *Journal of Speech and Hearing Research, 15*, 84-92.

Silverman, E.-M. (1973). Clustering: A characteristic of preschoolers' speech disfluency. *Journal of Speech and Hearing Research, 16*, 578-583.

Smith, A. (1990). Toward a comprehensive theory of stuttering: A commentary. *Journal of Speech and Hearing Disorders, 55*, 398-401.

St. Louis, K.O., & Westbrook, J. (1987). *The effectiveness of treatment for stuttering.* In L. Rustin, H. Purser, & D. Rowley (Eds.), *Progress in the treatment of fluency disorders.* London: Taylor and Francis.

St. Louis, K.O., & Lass, N.J. (1981). A survey of communicative disorders: Students' attitudes towards stuttering. *Journal of Fluency Disorders, 6*, 49-79.

St. Louis, K.O., Clausell, P.L., Thompson, J.N., & Rife, C.C. (1982). Preliminary investigation of EMG biofeedback induced relaxation with a preschool aged stutterer. *Perceptual and Motor Skills, 55*, 195-199.

Starkweather, C.W. (1982). Stuttering and laryngeal behavior: A review. *ASHA Monographs, 21.*

Starkweather, C.W. (1984). A multiprocess behavioral approach to stuttering therapy. In W.H. Perkins (Ed.), *Stuttering disorders.* New York: Thieme-Strattton.

Starkweather, C.W. (1987). *Fluency and stuttering.* Englewood Cliffs, New Jersey: Prentice Hall.

Starkweather, C.W. (1990). Current trends in therapy for stuttering children and suggestions for future research. *ASHA Reports, 18*, 82-90.

Starkweather, C.W., & Gottwald, S.R. (1990). The demands and capacities model II: Clinical applications. *Journal of Fluency Disorders, 15*, 143-157.

Starkweather, C.W., Gottwald, S. R. (1993). A pilot study of relations among specific measures obtained at intake and discharge in a program of prevention and early intervention for stuttering. *American Journal of Speech-Language Pathology, 2, 51-58.*

Starkweather, C.W., Gottwald, S.R., & Halfond, M.M. (1990). *Stuttering prevention: A clinical method.* Englewood Cliffs, NJ: Prentice Hall.

Starkweather, C.W., & Myers, M. (1979). Duration of subsegments within the intervocalic intervals in stutterers and nonstutterers. *Journal of Fluency Disorders, 4*, 205-214.

Stephenson-Opsal, D., & Ratner, N.B. (1988). Maternal speech rate modification and childhood stuttering. *Journal of Fluency Disorders, 13*, 49-56.

Stewart, J. (1985). Stuttering Indians: A reply to Zimmerman et al. *Journal of Speech and Hearing Research, 28*, 313-315.

Stocker, B., & Gerstman, L.J. (1983). A comparison of the probe technique and conventional therapy for young stutterers. *Journal of Fluency Disorders, 8*, 331-339.

Stokes, T.F., & Baer, D.M. (1977). An implicit technology of generalization. *Journal of Applied Behavior Analysis, 10*, 349-367.

Summers, J. (1986). Handwriting therapy: A possible tool for the speech therapist. *The Grapevine,* October/November.

Travis, L.E. (1931). *Speech Pathology.* New York: Appleton-Century.

Travis, L.E. (1986) Emotional factors. In G.H. Shames & H. Rubin (Eds.), *Stuttering then and now.* Columbus: Charles E. Merrill.

Travis, L.E. (1971). The unspeakable feelings of people with special reference to stuttering. In L.E. Travis (Ed.), *Handbook of speech pathology and audiology* . Englewood Cliffs, N.J.: Prentice-Hall.

Turnbaugh, K., & Guitar, B. (1981). Short-term intensive treatment in a public school setting. *Language, Speech, and Hearing Services in the Schools, 12*, 107-114.

Turpin, G. (1983). The behavioural management of tic-disorders: A critical review. *Advances in Behaviour Research and Therapy, 5*, 203-245.

Ulliana, L., & Ingham, R.J. (1984) Behavioral and nonbehavioral variables in the measurement of stutterers' communication attitudes. *Journal of Speech and Hearing Disorders, 49*, 83-93.

Van Riper, C. (1971). *The nature of stuttering.* Englewood Cliffs, N.J.: Prentice-Hall.

Van Riper, C. (1973). *The treatment of stuttering.* Englewood Cliffs, N.J.:Prentice-Hall.

Van Riper, C. (1982). *The Nature of Stuttering* (2nd. Ed.). Englewood Cliffs, NJ: Prentice-Hall.

Van Riper, C. (1992). Stuttering? *Journal of Fluency Disorders, 17*, 81-84..

Wall, M.J., & Myers, F.L. (1984). *Clinical management of childhood stuttering.* Baltimore: University Park Press.

Watson, B.C., & Alfonso, P.J. (1982). A comparison of LRT and VOT values between stutterers and nonstutterers. *Journal of Fluency Disorders, 7*, 219-241.

Watson, J.B. (1988). Profiles of stutterers' and nonstutterers' affective, cognitive, and behavioral communication attitudes. *Journal of Fluency Disorders, 12*, 389-405.

Weber, C., & Smith, A. (1990). Autonomic correlates of stuttering and speech assessed in a range of experimental tasks. *Journal of Speech and Hearing Research, 33*, 690-706.

Webster, R.L. (1980). Evolution of a target-based therapy for stuttering. *Journal of Fluency Disorders, 5*, 303-320.

Webster, R.L, & Lubker, B.B. (1968). Masking of auditory feedback in stutterers' speech. *Journal of Speech and Hearing Research, 11*, 221-223.

Webster, R.L., Morgan, B. T., & Cannon, M. W. (1987). Voice onset abruptness in stutterers before and after therapy. In H.F.M. Peters & W. Hulstijn (Eds.), *Speech Motor Dynamics and Stuttering.* New York: Springer-Verlag.

Weiss, A.L., & Zebrowski, P.M. (1992). Disfluencies in the conversations of young children who stutter: Some answers about questions. *Journal of Speech and Hearing Research, 35*, 1230-1238.

Wendahl, R.W., & Cole, J. (1961). Identification of stuttering during relatively fluent speech. *Journal of Speech and Hearing Research, 4*, 281-286.

West, R. (1958). An agnostic's speculations about stuttering. In J. Eisenson (Ed.), *Stuttering: A symposium.* New York: Harper and Row.

Westby, C. (1974). Language performance of stuttering and nonstuttering children. *Journal of Communication Disorders, 12*, 133-145.

Wexler, K., & Mysak, E. (1982). Disfluency characteristics of 2-, 4-, and 6-yr-old males. *Journal of Fluency Disorders, 7*, 37-46.

Williams, D.E. (1984). Prevention of stuttering. In W. H. Perkins (Ed.), *Stuttering disorders*. New York: Thieme-Stratton.

Williams, D.E., Silverman, F.H., & Kools, J.A. (1968). Disfluency behavior of elementary-school stutterers and nonstutterers: The adaptation effect. *Journal of Speech and Hearing Research, 11,* 662-630.

Wingate, M.E. (1964). A standard definition of stuttering. *Journal of Speech and Hearing Disorders, 29,* 484-489.

Wingate, M.E. (1969). Sound and pattern in "artificial" fluency.*Journal of Speech and Hearing Research, 12,* 677-686.

Wingate, M.E. (1970). The effect on stuttering of changes in audition.*Journal of Speech and Hearing Research, 13,* 861-873.

Wingate, M.E. (1971). The fear of stuttering. *Asha, 13,* 3-5.

Wingate, M.E. (1976). *Stuttering: Theory and treatment.* New York: Irvington.

Wingate, M.E. (1983). Speaking unassisted: Comments on a paper by Andrews et al. *Journal of Speech and Hearing Disorders, 48,* 255-263.

Wingate, M.E. (1984). Definition is the problem. *Journal of Speech and Hearing Disorders, 49,* 429-431.

Wingate, M.E. (1988). *Stuttering: A psycholinguistic analysis.* New York: Springer-Verlag.

Winkler, L.E., & Ramig, P. (1986). Temporal characteristics in the fluent speech of child stutterers and nonstutterers. *Journal of Fluency Disorders, 11,* 217-229.

Wischner, G. (1950). Stuttering behavior and learning: A preliminary theoretical formulation. *Journal of Speech and Hearing Disorders, 15,* 324-335.

Wischner, G.J. (1952). Anxiety-reduction as reinforcement in maladaptive behavior: Evidence in stutterers' representations of the moment of difficulty. *Journal of Abnormal Social Psychology, 47,* 566-571.

Woolf, G. (1967). The assessment of stuttering as struggle, avoidance, and expectancy. *British Journal of Disorders of Communication, 2,* 158-171.

World Health Organization (1977). *Manual of the international statistical classification of diseases, injuries, and causes of death* (Vol. 1). Geneva: World Health Organization.

Yairi, E. (1981). Disfluencies of normally speaking two-year-old children. *Journal of Speech and Hearing Research, 24,* 490-495.

Yairi, E. (1982). Longitudinal studies of disfluencies in two-year old children. *Journal of Speech and Hearing Research, 25,* 155-160.

Yairi, E. (1983). The onset of stuttering in two- and three-year-old children: A preliminary report. *Journal of Speech and Hearing Disorders, 48,* 171-177.

Yairi, E., & Ambrose, N. (1992a). Onset of stuttering in preschool children: Selected factors. *Journal of Speech and Hearing Research, 35,* 782-788.

Yairi, E., & Ambrose, N. (1992b). A longitudinal study of stuttering in children: A preliminary report. *Journal of Speech and Hearing Research, 35,* 755-760.

Yairi, E., Ambrose, N., & Niermann, R. (1993). The early months of stuttering: A developmental study. *Journal of Speech and Hearing Research, 36,* 521-528.

Yairi, E., & Clifton, N.F. (1972). Disfluent speech behavior of preschool children, high school seniors, and geriatric persons. *Journal of Speech and Hearing Research, 15,* 714-719.

Yairi, E., & Lewis, B. (1984) Disfluencies at the onset of stuttering.*Journal of Speech and Hearing Research, 27,* 154-159.

Yaruss & Conture xx Insert reference

Yeudall, L.T. (1985). A neuro-psychological theory of stuttering. *Seminars in Speech and Language, 6,* 197-231

Young, M.A. (1964). Identification of stutterers from recorded samples of their "fluent speech." *Journal of Speech and Hearing Research, 7,* 302-303.

Young, M.A. (1975a). Onset, prevalence, and recovery from stuttering. *Journal of Speech and Hearing Disorders, 40,* 49-58.

Young, M.A. (1975b). Observer agreement for marking moments of stuttering. *Journal of Speech and Hearing Research, 18,* 530-540.

Young, M.A. (1981). A reanalysis of "Stuttering therapy: The relationship between attitude change and long-term outcome". *Journal of Speech and Hearing Disorders, 46,* 221-222.

Young, M.A. (1984). Identification of stuttering and stutterers. In R.F. Curlee & W.H. Perkins (Eds.) *Nature and treatment of stuttering: New directions.* San Diego: College-Hill Press.

Zebrowski, P. (1991). Duration of the speech disfluencies of beginning stutterers. *Journal of Speech and Hearing Research, 34,* 483-491.

Zebrowski, P.M., & Conture, E.G. (1989). Judgements of disfluency by mothers of stuttering and normally fluent children.*Journal of Speech and Hearing Research, 32*, 625-634.

Zebrowski, P.M., Conture, E.G. & Cudahy, E.A. (1985). Acoustic analysis of young stutterers' fluency: Preliminary observations. *Journal of Fluency Disorders, 10*, 173-192.

Zimmermann, G. (1980). Stuttering: A disorder of movement. *Journal of Speech and Hearing Research, 23*, 108-121.

Zimmermann, G. (1984). Articulatory dynamics of stutterers. In R.F. Curlee and W.H. Perkins (Eds.). *Nature and treatment of stuttering: New directions.* San Diego: College-Hill Press.

Zimmermann, G., & Hanley, J. (1983). A cinefluorographic investigation of repeated fluent productions of stutterers in an adaptation procedure. *Journal of Speech and Hearing Research, 26*, 35-42.

Zimmermann, G., Liljeblad, S., Frank, A., & Cleeland, C. (1983). The Indians have many terms for it: Stuttering among the Bannock-Shoshoni. *Journal of Speech and Hearing Research, 26*, 315-318.

Zimmermann, G., Smith, A., & Hanley, J. (1981). Stuttering: In need of a unifying conceptual framework. *Journal of Speech and Hearing Research, 46*, 25-31.

# Index